Praise for
Creating & Sustaining Civility in Nursing Education, Second Edition

"The positive impact of this book is possible because of the tremendous passion and commitment that Cindy Clark has for creating healthy work environments. Conversations about incivility can be challenging because they often touch people in a very personal and emotional way; however, Clark manages to discuss civility in a respectful yet realistic manner. Clark masterfully shares aspects of her own journey as well as stories from many leaders, nurse educators, and students. She discusses tools and strategies that can be implemented to address the problem of incivility, offering encouragement and hope. This book is a must have for leaders and educators in academia and clinical practice to promote civility in nursing education."

–Sheryl Sommer, PhD, RN, CNE
Vice President and Chief Nursing Officer
ATI Nursing Education

"Clark's book should be a required text for every master's student in education and/or leadership in nursing education. It is destined to become dog-eared and highlighted as it is read and reread over time. Cindy demonstrates how to blend evidence-based research findings with anecdotes and musings, in a fascinating, alternately heartbreaking and uplifting read. It reads as if you are talking with a buddy walking along a mountain path, or on the beach, or in an aspen grove."

–Suzan "Suzie" Kardong-Edgren, PhD, RN, ANEF, CHSE, FAAN
Professor and RISE Center Director, School of Nursing and Health Sciences,
Robert Morris University
Adjunct Associate Professor, Drexel Graduate School of Biomedical Sciences
and Professional Studies College of Medicine

"Cindy Clark has helped us understand the issue and impact of incivility in nursing and nursing education. The second edition of *Creating and Sustaining Civility in Nursing Education* is a must-read book for all nurse educators, administrators, and graduate students preparing for a role as an educator. A strength of this book is its blending of research with practical tips for creating a positive learning environment for students."

–Marilyn H. Oermann, PhD, RN, ANEF, FAAN
Thelma M. Ingles Professor of Nursing, Duke University School of Nursing
Editor-in-Chief of Nurse Educator

"What Dr. Clark has created is a sustained and impassioned call for action to address one of the most difficult problems we face across our lives through an appreciative framework of civility. Her comprehensive approach across the workforce and education settings recognizes the complexity of the issues we face and the integrative solutions needed to prevent and address bullying in education and practice settings. Her sharing of her personal story and her ability to give practical solutions that translate easily into the real world are gifts that can lift others up to meet the challenge. A must-read for those in education and practice, but even more a book whose lessons must be lived."

–*Cole Edmonson, DNP, RN, FACHE, NEA-BC, FAAN*
Chief Nursing Officer
Texas Health Dallas

"Through this exquisite book, Clark has given us a great gift. The personal experiences, heart-wrenching stories of far too many faculty and students, and research findings are profound, and they challenge readers to reflect on our own behaviors, honestly and openly. The wise strategies offered by Clark, however, help us realize that we can and must act to create communities of civility in our academic environments and not just shake our heads about "the way the world is today." This is a book that every nurse educator should read with the intention of monitoring and changing, as needed, our own behaviors and the culture of the communities in which we practice as teachers in order to create positive learning environments with students and healthful, civil work environments with faculty colleagues."

–*Theresa M. "Terry" Valiga, EdD, RN, CNE, ANEF, FAAN*
Professor; Director, Institute for Educational Excellence; and
Chair, Division of Clinical Systems and Analytics
Duke University School of Nursing

"Cindy Clark's second edition is an absolute must-read. Cindy is a nationally renowned expert in best strategies to create and sustain civility in order to achieve great outcomes in nursing education and the workplace. Once you read this book, you will have evidence-based tactics to put into practice in creating an optimal and healthy work environment."

–*Bernadette Mazurek Melnyk, PhD, RN, CPNP/PMHNP, FAANP, FNAP,*
FAAN
Associate Vice President for Health Promotion, University Chief Wellness
Officer
Dean and Professor, College of Nursing, and Professor of Pediatrics &
Psychiatry, College of Medicine
The Ohio State University
President, the National Consortium for Building Healthy Academic
Communities (NCBHAC)
Editor, Worldviews on Evidence-based Nursing

"Frankly, I did not think the first edition of this text could be topped, but Dr. Clark has indeed found a way to go above and beyond to create a masterful, cogent, and impactful book that I consider to be the definitive work on this topic. She is without a doubt one of the freshest, most reflective, and introspective thinkers on the topic of incivility in healthcare and nursing academia, and she does not shy away from exploring this complex topic from a variety of perspectives. Using her own and others' compelling stories as well as the most relevant and contemporary research to inform us, she completely deconstructs the topic of incivility in nursing education. More importantly, she tackles it in such a way that the reader is left not only hopeful, but inspired, energized, and empowered to cultivate civility in his or her own surroundings. And, with renewed focus on achievable, real-life solutions, this updated edition will prove to be a highly useful guide to those who share her vision for creating civil learning environments where all can thrive. Clark's compelling work has the potential to radically alter nursing and nursing education as we know it—for the better!"

–Susan Luparell, PhD, RN, CNE, ANEF
Associate Professor
Montana State University College of Nursing

"This seminal book on creating civility in nursing education is well-written, comprehensive, and scholarly. Readers will enjoy the personal approach and illustrative cases that are integrated throughout, as well as the many interactive exercises and self-assessments. I am impressed with the amount of evidence presented that clearly supports the issue of incivility in nursing education as a troubling problem. Not only does it affect the individual being bullied, but it also adversely affects patient safety and even impacts the regulation of nursing programs. Clark then presents many research-based and user-friendly strategies for creating a civilized environment, addressing diverse audiences, including students, faculty, and organizations. This book is a must-read for nurse educators and administrators, practitioners, regulators, and students."

–Nancy Spector, PhD, RN, FAAN
Director Regulatory Innovations
National Council of State Boards of Nursing

"When we use the word 'powerful' with the concept of incivility, we think of someone or something that can stop someone acting out. We may conjure up the tall adult hovering over a child and saying 'stop it!' We may see someone giving 'the look' (which also means 'stop it!'). Now we can envision the great blue heron. I have admired Cindy and her work for years, and yes, somehow I missed the first edition of this book. That was my loss. Let me tell you why.

When we think of reading about civility and incivility, we may think about dry, boring statistics, a few poignant stories, and long, convoluted sentences. If that is what you expect here, you are wrong! From the beginning introduction to the last word of text, Cindy has written with the grace of a best-selling author. Her words paint pictures that allow us to see a situation and experience the emotions of that situation. If you don't see yourself in at least one situation, you haven't been paying attention to life! Because of her well-established expertise on this topic, we also find truth; and the truth will lead us to resolution—or at least improvement.

The book reads like a novel and yet includes a considerable amount of documented research, often that of her and her colleagues, on the topic. Further, the book is peppered with civility tips, which are practical strategies designed to enhance our practice of being civil. While the title references nursing education and the examples are faculty and students, insightful readers can see that these situations occur in other fields and in other work settings, including those in healthcare. Additionally, Cindy includes several civility index tools so that anyone can learn more about his/her personal behavior. Her expertise shines through the strategies offered to deal with difficult challenges. She inspires us to actively seek out incivility and address it proactively—for the benefit of the aggressor and the recipient of uncivil behavior. This book is one of those that will remain prominently displayed on a nearby bookshelf because it will be referenced frequently. Uncivil behavior is not a one-shot deal, and neither is correcting that behavior. Cindy provides us with the road map for ourselves and our organizations."

–Patricia S. Yoder-Wise, EdD, RN, NEA-BC, ANEF, FAAN
Dean Emerita and Professor Emerita,
Texas Tech University Health Sciences Center School of Nursing
President, The Wise Group

Creating & Sustaining Civility in Nursing Education

Second Edition

Cynthia Clark, PhD, RN, ANEF, FAAN

Sigma Theta Tau International
Honor Society of Nursing®

> The Honor Society of Nursing, Sigma Theta Tau International (STTI) is a nonprofit organization founded in 1922 whose mission is advancing world health and celebrating nursing excellence in scholarship, leadership, and service. Members include practicing nurses, instructors, researchers, policymakers, entrepreneurs, and others. STTI has 512 chapters located at more than 700 institutions of higher education throughout Armenia, Australia, Botswana, Brazil, Canada, Colombia, England, Ghana, Hong Kong, Japan, Kenya, Lebanon, Malawi, Mexico, the Netherlands, Pakistan, Philippines, Portugal, Singapore, South Africa, South Korea, Swaziland, Sweden, Taiwan, Tanzania, Thailand, the United Kingdom, and the United States of America. More information about STTI can be found online at www.nursingsociety.org.

Sigma Theta Tau International
550 West North Street
Indianapolis, IN, USA 46202

To order additional books, buy in bulk, or order for corporate use, contact Nursing Knowledge International at 888.NKI.4YOU (888.654.4968/US and Canada) or +1.317.634.8171 (outside US and Canada).

To request a review copy for course adoption, email solutions@nursingknowledge.org or call 888. NKI.4YOU (888.654.4968/US and Canada) or +1.317.634.8171 (outside US and Canada).

To request author information, or for speaker or other media requests, contact Marketing, Honor Society of Nursing, Sigma Theta Tau International at 888.634.7575 (US and Canada) or +1.317.634.8171 (outside US and Canada).

ISBN: 9781945157059
EPUB ISBN: 9781945157066
PDF ISBN: 9781945157073
MOBI ISBN: 9781945157080

Clark, Cynthia M. (Cynthia Marie), author. | Sigma Theta Tau
 International, issuing body.
Creating & sustaining civility in nursing education / Cynthia Clark.
Creating and sustaining civility in nursing education
Second edition. | Indianapolis : Sigma Theta Tau International,
 [2017] | Includes bibliographical references and index.
LCCN 2016045512 (print) | LCCN 2016046510 (ebook) | ISBN
 9781945157059 (print : alk. paper) | ISBN 9781945157066 (epub) | ISBN
 9781945157073 (pdf) | ISBN 9781945157080 (mobi) | ISBN 9781945157066
 (Epub) | ISBN 9781945157073 (Pdf) | ISBN 9781945157080 (Mobi)
 | MESH: Education, Nursing | Students, Nursing--psychology |
 Interprofessional Relations--ethics | Leadership
LCC RT85 (print) | LCC RT85 (ebook) | NLM WY 18 | DDC
 610.73--dc23
LC record available at https://lccn.loc.gov/2016045512

First Printing, 2017

Publisher: Dustin Sullivan   Principal Book Editor: Carla Hall
Acquisitions Editor: Emily Hatch   Content & Project Editor: Kevin Kent
Editorial Coordinator: Paula Jeffers   Copy Editor: Erin Geile
Cover Designer: Kim Scott   Proofreader: Todd Lothery
Interior Design/Page Layout: Katy Bodenmiller   Indexer: Larry Sweazy

Dedication

I dedicate this book to the thousands of students, faculty members, academic and practice-based nurse leaders, and healthcare professionals who have bravely shared their stories with me—often heart-wrenching encounters with incivility—and, in many cases, their subsequent triumph over these difficult experiences. I offer this book to nurse educators and nurses across the globe who work tirelessly every day to prepare, educate, and inspire our nursing workforce and who kindle the flame for nursing practice, leadership, scholarship, policy change, and activism.

Acknowledgments

If you have attended one of my civility presentations, you know I always start each session expressing appreciation by thanking the participants for sharing part of their busy day with me. I am honored by their presence and grateful for their attendance. It seems equally fitting that I begin this book by expressing gratitude.

First, a thank you to the chorus of many wise women in my life:

To my mother and grandmother, who loved me completely and unconditionally. They instilled in me a genuine sense of respect for others and emphasized the importance of service. Not only did they stress the principles of civility and social justice, they lived them every day. To my mother-in-law, an enduring and impressive role model; leading by example, she lives an examined, purposeful, and meaningful life.

To Dr. Hildegard Messenbaugh, who taught me and so many others how to be accomplished and compassionate clinicians as well as better people, always stressing the importance of the three Rs: relationships, relationships, and relationships—constantly reminding us that it is and always will be the people in our lives who matter most.

To Dr. Anne Payne, who took a risk by hiring me so many years ago. She saw something special in a young, would-be nursing professor when others couldn't or wouldn't. And to my early mentor, Pat Taylor, who showed me how to navigate and appreciate the intricacies of higher education and to always keep students front and center. And in recent years, my gratitude to Dr. Pam Springer for her support for my work and unwavering generosity. Pam's mentorship and friendship are treasures indeed.

A grand bouquet of gratitude to my friends and colleagues at ATI Nursing Education, who have given me the amazing opportunity to collaborate with nurses, students, faculty, and healthcare professionals across the country to transform workplaces and to ultimately make the world a better place for all of us—especially the patients entrusted with our care.

I am grateful to my colleagues and friends at Boise State University— as a loyal and an avid fan of the "Blue," I wish to express my ardent appreciation to the individuals who have contributed to this work.

Thank you to Drs. Kathleen Heinrich and Susan Luparell; I will always cherish the "safe place" we co-created to discuss and unfold the myriad complexities of incivility and to identify creative ways to address the problem.

A great, big, magnificent thank you and "shout out" to Dr. Diane Billings, a role model and mentor extraordinaire, who epitomizes civility and grace of the highest order.

A very special thank you to the many contributors to this book, far too many to name, but each of you know who you are. I am forever grateful to you for sharing your ideas, stories, and pearls of wisdom that have clearly made this book a much better product.

This book would not have been possible without the expertise and unwavering support I received from my acquiring editor, Emily Hatch. You promised to walk with me every step of the way on this journey, and never once did you fail to keep your word. I am forever grateful to you for your responsiveness, kindness, and unyielding belief in me. To Carla Hall and Kevin Kent, editors extraordinaire: Thank you for your thoughtful and inspiring comments and suggestions. You have made this book so much better. Jim Mattson, you continue to be an incredible source of inspiration. Your kindness and decency are gifts that keep on giving, and I will always be grateful for encouragement to author the first edition of this book by quoting John Bytheway, who quipped, "Inch by inch, life's a cinch." You have no idea how many times that quote kept me centered and moving along one inch and one word at a time!

A special thank you to my beloved furry friends, our cherished crew of shelter pets. You were with me as I crafted each sentence, paragraph, and page of this book, and you listened patiently and without criticism as I read passages aloud to seek your opinions. As the saying goes, I wonder, "Who rescued whom?" Thanks for being my faithful friends!

And lastly, to my husband, Greg, my best friend, the love of my life, and my soulmate—thank you! When we met as young undergraduates more than 35 years ago, who knew we would become the parents of three awesome, productive, and beautiful children and that you would always be the joy of my life, my biggest fan, and the greatest husband a woman could ever have. I love you beyond measure.

About the Author

Cynthia Clark, PhD, RN, ANEF, FAAN, is an award-winning, tenured professor, professor emeritus, and strategic nursing advisor for ATI Nursing Education. As a clinician, she specialized in adolescent mental health, substance abuse intervention and recovery, and violence prevention. She is the founder of Civility Matters™ and a leading expert in fostering civility and healthy work environments. In 2015, she served as a co-chair for the American Nurses Association Professional Panel for Incivility, Bullying, and Workplace Violence. Her groundbreaking work on fostering civility has brought national and international attention to the controversial issues of incivility in academic and work environments. Her theory-driven interventions, empirical measurements, theoretical models, and reflective assessments provide "best practices" to prevent, measure, and address uncivil behavior and to create healthy workplaces.

Clark serves as a fellow in the American Academy of Nursing and the National League for Nursing Academy of Nursing Education. Her presentations number in the hundreds and her publications have appeared in a broad range of peer-reviewed and open-access venues. She is the recipient of numerous teaching, research, and service awards including the 2011 and 2012 Most Inspirational Professor Award, the 2011 NLN Excellence in Educational Research Award, and the 2013 *Journal of Nursing Education* (JNE) Christine A. Tanner Scholary Writing Award. The first edition of her book, *Creating and Sustaining Civility in Nursing Education*, received first-place honors as the 2013 *American Journal of Nursing* Book of the Year for Professional Issues in Nursing. She has been a member of the Honor Society of Nursing, Sigma Theta Tau International (STTI) for more than two decades and has served STTI in numerous capacities, including her contributions as a professional blogger for *Reflections on Nursing Leadership* since 2010.

Clark's research involves preparing nursing students, faculty, and practice-based nurses to prevent and address incivility in academic and healthcare settings; bridging the gap between nursing education and practice-based nurses to foster healthy work environments; addressing student stress, coping, and pursuance of academic civility; and ongoing intervention studies, including a biomarker study to measure the effectiveness of cognitive rehearsal as a means to mitigate stress and protect patient safety following uncivil encounters. Her empirical instruments to measure incivility and promote civility have been translated into several languages and have been used to conduct studies in the United States, Israel, Iran, Indonesia, the Philippines, the People's Republic of China, Malaysia, Jordan, Canada, Uganda, Korea, Saudi Arabia, Nigeria, and Ecuador. She has served as a committee member and content expert for several graduate student studies, both nationally and internationally; many have used her empirical instruments in their doctoral dissertations, master's theses, and other scholarly works.

Clark is also well-known for her expertise in the area of scholarly teaching, learner-centered pedagogies, and active learning strategies. For several years, she has used live theater actors, simulation, and student-produced YouTube videos as active learning strategies to promote student engagement and deep learning. In her role as a teaching scholar for faculty learning communities, Clark facilitated the development of several early-career faculty members in their growth as scholarly educators and learner-centered teachers, and has conducted numerous classroom observations and assessments to help faculty improve their pedagogical approaches.

She spends her leisure time kickboxing, hiking, biking, cooking, and reading. She especially enjoys spending time with her family and pets. For more information about Clark and her work on f ostering civility, please visit her Civility Matters website at http://hs.boisestate.edu/civilitymatters/ and her *Musing of the Great Blue* blog, published by STTI, at http://musingofthegreatblue.blogspot.com/.

Table of Contents

Foreword

In the first edition of *Creating & Sustaining Civility*, Cynthia Clark challenged nurses, nurse educators, and students to make civility a priority. Yet, in spite of the availability of tools to assess student, faculty, and organizational civility; guidance about how to create a culture of civility; and workshops to prepare nurses for their responsibilities in sustaining civility, findings from recent studies continue to reveal unacceptable levels of incivility in nursing and nursing education. The second edition of Clark's book is compelling and timely, offering both action plans and hope along with best practices for fostering civility and healthy work and academic environments where individuals can thrive and achieve their greatest potential.

In this edition, readers will find additional evidence-based tools and strategies to promote civility in online and on-campus classrooms and in the academic and practice workplace. Clark has placed increased emphasis on ethics and has included key information stemming from position papers of professional nursing organizations, such as ANA's position statement on Incivility, Bullying, and Workplace Violence. New scenarios provide examples of how to manage conflict and effectively address and negotiate uncivil encounters. Learn-at-a glance sidebars and tables present succinct tips for developing respectful personal and organizational communication. Revised conceptual models explicate the intertwined relationships between nursing practice and nursing education and their joint responsibilities for fostering civility.

As Clark advises us, civility begins with understanding and managing factors that contribute to uncivil behavior; articulating norms of civil behavior and aligning them with policies and procedures; establishing a civility team to oversee implementation of plans; and empowering *civility champions*, crusaders dedicated to improving civility in our schools of nursing and healthcare organizations. Also important are assessing the organizational culture on an ongoing basis and ensuring that during the admission or hiring processes and subsequent orientation, the values for civil encounters and behavioral expectations are clearly articulated and upheld. This book provides all the resources you and your organization need to create and sustain civility and to foster healthy work environments.

As nurses, we are on the front line of creating and sustaining a civil and just society. This is a time for hope and optimism, and now, more than ever, we owe it to our patients, students, and colleagues to lead by creating a pathway toward civility. Let Clark, at her teacher-author best, help you learn how.

—*Diane M. Billings, EdD, RN, FAAN, ANEF*
Chancellor's Professor of Nursing
Indiana University School of Nursing, Indianapolis

Introduction

When I was a child, I dreamed of growing up to be a major league baseball player. Specifically, my goal was to play second base for the Chicago Cubs. Cheering for the Boys in Blue with the other zany bleacher bums, surrounded by the ivy-covered walls of Wrigley Field on opening day, I was inspired to fulfill my dream. Someday, I would be a player adding to the joy and excitement of America's favorite pastime. Until then, while growing up in farm country, my summer jobs included detasseling corn, de-rouging bean fields, and dip painting machine parts for tomato harvesters. Great work if you can get it! But a funny thing happened on the way to the ballpark. The summer of my senior year in high school, the parents of my best friend (a physician and a nurse), who owned a long-term care center, asked if I would like a job working as a nurse's aide. This decision—as many do—would change the course and direction of my life and fade the ambitions of my baseball career.

I'll never forget my first day as a nurse's aide. Back then, we were trained on the job by the unit charge nurse. Imagine my immense surprise when my charge nurse (Nurse Grey) turned out to be the same nurse who was in the delivery room with my mother the day I was born. She was a force! A large, imposing woman both in stature and presence. She took one look at me and said, "I remember you like it was yesterday. You certainly were a homely one." That was the introduction to my first day on the job. But in the end, I learned more about myself and caring for others than I ever thought possible. These powerful lessons learned during adolescence as a young nurse's aide formed an enduring and lasting impression that would ultimately shape my eventual nursing career.

Nurse Grey and other members of the team took me under their collective and compassionate wing. Through their tutelage, they taught me many important aspects of nursing. Yet ultimately, it was the residents from whom I learned some of the most impressive and important lessons in my life. Even today, when I close my eyes and picture the residents living in the east wing, I can recall their names, faces, habits, preferences, and, most of all, their stories.

I'd like to share one of the stories with you. It's a bit of a love story, although not the type of love story that typically comes to mind. Instead, this story is about a teenager (me) who grew to love an elderly resident at the assisted living center. His name was Albert. I didn't know it at the time, but Albert would change the course of my life. He would eventually teach me some profound lessons about caring, about compassion, about living, and about dying.

I first met Albert when I was assigned to his care as a young nurse's aide. As a younger man, Albert had been severely injured in a construction accident, leaving him an amputee and wheelchair bound. In more recent years, he had suffered a stroke that threatened to weaken him, but he fought the good fight and refused to yield to the physical limitations and the compromise of his condition. I loved his spirit and his tenacity. The highlight of my working day was spending time with him, listening to his stories and recounting the history of his life. Each day was a journey into the existence of a man who loved life, cherished his family, and feared little. Every day I looked forward to our conversations. He taught me to believe in goodness and kindness and challenged me to dream big and in living color. He encouraged me by example to make a difference in the world and to leave a footprint on this earth—a footprint that would be indelible and one I would be proud to leave. He inspired me to reach higher than I ever believed I could, and he encouraged me to become a nurse. He loved nurses, he loved the profession, and I know he loved me.

As an adolescent I gave little thought to my future, but I listened to Albert and what he said about the journey of life and its many twists and turns. I took note of his lessons, and they all mattered deeply to me. One day, I arrived at work, and I saw the ambulance pulling away. I knew from experience that one of the residents had died, and I wondered who it might be. I entered the building, and the night nurse embraced me. She hugged me tightly and whispered softly that Albert had died quietly and peacefully during the night with his beautiful wife of 50 years by his side. I was devastated by the news. Yet, it was a crystalizing event in my life and a defining moment for my future career. I decided then that I would become a nurse, and make a difference, and leave that much-discussed and highly cherished footprint.

Albert was one of my role models and one of my most treasured heroes. He inspired me to lead a mindful and purposeful life—to live a life that matters and to promise to make a difference. One of the most important ways for me to fulfill this promise was to share my experiences and stories with others. So, when I was approached by the publishing branch of Sigma Theta Tau International in the spring of 2012, asking if I might be interested in authoring a book about fostering civility in nursing education, this was an opportunity I could not ignore. I remember taking the phone call as I looked out the big bay window of our beloved country home, gazing at the high desert and the rolling hills of Southwest Idaho, surrounded by several mountain ranges inhabited by herds of deer, antelope, and elk. The view helped center me. At first, I was surprised by the request; then, after giving it the deliberation that such a decision deserves, I was excited to share my thoughts on civility with my fellow nurse educators across the country and around the globe. Since the release of the first edition of this book, I have been blessed with an overwhelmingly positive response and expression of gratitude for providing a valuable resource to prevent and address incivility and to build communities of civility across the country and throughout the world. It's an exhilarating yet deeply humbling experience.

So, when Emily Hatch, the acquiring editor for STTI, called me to suggest a second edition of *Creating and Sustaining Civility in Nursing Education,* I found myself physically, emotionally, and spiritually migrating to the same space that I had occupied the first time I spoke with Emily about publishing a book on civility. It was a beautiful spring day in 2016. I looked out that same big bay window and took in the high-desert scenery of Idaho, surrounded by mountains and deep blue skies. The trees were beginning to bud and the sun was shining brilliantly. Our myriad band of rescue pets were lazily sunning on the back deck without a care in the world. I stood there on purpose, centering myself as I considered the importance of continuing to carry the message of civility and healthy work environments to others. I realize that the fire to inspire, and the passion to lead the coalition to create and sustain communities of civility, burns hotter and more intense than ever. It is my fervent desire to share evidence-based solutions and promising practices to improve lives and to foster healthy work and learning environments that promote dignity for all and embody the principles of civility, professionalism, and ethical conduct. Without question, it is simply the right thing to do. I took a deep breath and said *yes,* let's do it.

In this edition, the focus remains on creating a product that is readable and conversational—a book that faculty will read, use, and reuse. My hope is that this book will appeal to aspiring and seasoned nursing faculty at all levels of nursing education. My intention is to inform and captivate the reader in a highly engaging manner. I have included stories, exemplars, and tools to address the problem of incivility. But mostly, I hope to instill an enthusiasm to promote civility in nursing education—to fan the flames of respect and to sing civility from the rooftops.

As before, writing this edition was preceded each day by hiking to the top of the knoll outside our back door with a cup of coffee in hand and our five rescue pets in tow. I love walking through the early morning sunlight and breezes greeting the day and welcoming the world. We have "pausing points" along the hike, places where the pups and I look out over the blue skies and open spaces where horses graze and birds sing with joy for a new day—a wonderful way to "get my head in the game" before writing.

This book is intended to be used and reused. My goal is to provide an informative and valued resource and one with suggestions for fostering civility that can be implemented. The first part of the book includes reflections on incivility and civility, a description of the relationship between stress and incivility, and a comprehensive overview of civility and incivility in nursing education. The second part of the book presents a variety of evidence-based strategies that faculty can implement to promote civility and respect in nursing education. Strategies range from immediate, ready-to-use teaching tools to suggestions for leading and transforming broad-based institutional change.

Please accept this book as my gift to you—to nurse educators everywhere who greet each day with purpose and intention to make the world a better place. It contains a piece of my heart that you can carry with you as you pursue and achieve civility in your daily lives and in the lives of all those you and your students touch. Go forward Civility Champions, and enjoy the journey.

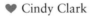 Cindy Clark

About the great blue heron image: This majestic bird is a beautiful, graceful, and noble creature—representing self-determination, self-reliance, patience, presence, and the innate wisdom necessary to co-create one's own circumstances. That's how I view pursuing civility. There are those among us who have the grace and nobility to speak the truth, the self-determination to transform and revolutionize the human condition, and the ability to use our innate wisdom to create and sustain cultures of civility and respect.

Chapter 1
Reflections on Incivility and Why Civility Matters

When we are on the receiving end of an act of civility, we feel validated, valued, and it gives our life meaning. –P. M. Forni

This chapter discusses:

- My civility story and the influence of wise women
- The imperative of civility
- How eye-rolling can escalate to tragedy

Growing Up Civil

I grew up near Chicago, the third of six children in a middle-class, hard-working, Irish Catholic family. I enjoyed a magical childhood filled with friends, family, and the great outdoors. Life was good and largely influenced by the formidable matriarchs of our family, especially my mother and maternal grandmother. Both taught me many important life lessons—and both were adamant about sending me and my five siblings to parochial schools. As a product of the Catholic school system, I was taught by Dominican nuns under the guidance of a strict monsignor who believed not only in the three Rs but also in deportment and character development. At the time I was not a big fan of being graded on such behaviors as "is courteous in speech and manner," "respects the rights of others," and "works and plays well with others." But believe me, our parents took these grades very seriously—often more seriously than our academic performance. Is it any wonder that civility and respect for others are central features in my body of research—and in my life?

My mother reinforced the importance of extending kindness and providing service to all creatures, both human and nonhuman, especially those most vulnerable, those who needed us most. I was encouraged to accept others without judgment and to leave the world a better place than I found it. She instilled in us an appreciation for standing for what's good and right, and she lived what she believed—that we must consider the legacy by which we hope to be remembered. What difference will we make in the world? What ignites our passion, and how is that passion sustained? For me, I am convinced that we each make a difference by doing the small and simple things in life that add value and improve the lives of those around us. Of course, this is an ongoing process, one never perfected, because in my humanity, I make and sometimes keep making the same mistakes. Yet I, like most of the readers who have picked up this book, strive to make a meaningful difference in the lives of those I encounter each day.

Having a grandmother and mother like mine left a lifelong impression, and consequently, respect, humility, and civility are part of my DNA. Uneducated in the formal sense, these wise women taught me lessons beyond the textbooks and lecture halls of the ivory tower. They taught me to smile more, to love deeper, and to pay it forward—to find my passion and use it to add meaning in the world and to inspire others to do the same.

As I left my childhood behind, I met and eventually married my husband of more than 30 years. When I met him, I was introduced to another influential woman, my mother-in-law, who was born in southern Virginia on a tobacco farm. She is a thoughtful, wise, and deeply reflective person. We have spent countless hours walking and talking—sharing our innermost thoughts about life, family, and our mutual love of the earth. She often shares her life philosophies with me, and we both spend time in quietness to listen to the voices of our soul, to examine the meaning of these inner voices, and to find and fulfill our purpose in life. Today, at the age of 94, my mother-in-law unfailingly inspires me with her enduring focus on healthy living, devotion to introspection, and attention to spiritual development and self-improvement.

Creating communities of civility and respect is my purpose and my calling. My professional mission includes being an outspoken and ardent leader for lasting change, creating and sustaining communities of civility, and inspiring healthy workplaces and positive relationships. My goal is to raise awareness about the existence and consequences of incivility, to amplify the national dialogue on fostering civil work and learning environments, and to be a role model and an ambassador for lasting change—in short, to lead and mobilize the coalition for change and to inspire *civility champions* for the civility movement. I must admit, however, that in the beginning of my nursing education, I doubted the integrity of the profession and deeply questioned my career choice. My experience as a young nursing student is a sad but all-too-common story. My personal experience with faculty incivility was a lengthy and painful one, but the story also contains examples of courage, compassion, and the power of relationships. It is a story with a happy ending, one that emphasizes the capacity of genuine caring and effective mentoring. The following story is excerpted from Clark (2010).

The Sweet Spot of Civility: My Story

As I entered my nursing education program, almost immediately I loved my new life, and I was definitely in my element...but only for a while. It did not take long before one of the nursing faculty (I'll call her Professor Sour) showed her true nature. She was a negative force indeed. As students, we feared Professor Sour as we all became targets of her belittling remarks and bullying behaviors. For some reason, which still perplexes me today, Professor Sour took a particular dislike toward me. Being only 18 years old, I was inexperienced and ill-equipped to deal with rude and demeaning teachers—or any adult, for that matter. I believed that my best defense was to fly under the radar and attempt to avoid her.

But that was easier said than done, because Professor Sour was a lead instructor for several of my classes, including my clinical experiences. Nevertheless, I tried without much success to stay on her good side, but inevitably she would find reasons to berate me, often in full view and in earshot of other students, nurses, physicians, and sometimes even patients. I kept thinking that sooner or later Professor Sour would grow tired of humiliating me, but unfortunately, she seemed to delight in tormenting me. My classmates were supportive, but they experienced the wrath of Professor Sour as well and tried to avoid her as much as I did. So I decided to power through the put-downs and try to ignore what seemed to be daily disrespectful and rude remarks.

That strategy was woefully ineffective, as the incivility grew and deepened. Professor Sour found unique ways to demean and degrade me, until her bullying behaviors hit new heights when she attempted to publicly embarrass me in front of several physicians and nurses when I asked to leave the clinical unit to use the restroom. I considered leaving the unit without her permission but quickly dismissed the thought, knowing that it would only further enrage her. So, I asked permission and was immediately rebuked and castigated by Professor Sour. There I stood in front of everyone, filled with the deep humiliation that only a teenager can feel when being publicly chastised and demeaned—especially about a private and personal matter. It wasn't until much later I realized that it was not I who suffered the greatest embarrassment that day; instead it was Professor Sour, who publicly humiliated and shamed a young nursing student who simply asked to use the restroom. It was a defining moment in my professional life and one that I have never forgotten.

You can probably imagine that I seriously considered leaving nursing school and pursuing another profession. However, even at the vulnerable age of 18, I had an internal strength—or maybe it was defiance—and I was not going to give up easily. The hostility from Professor Sour became even worse, though she managed to hide her harsh remarks from others. Her incivility was covert, and for a while her torment seemed to go unnoticed by others. But of course, I noticed, and the pain I experienced was profound and intense. When I dared to share my feelings and experiences with my classmates, they empathized and offered friendship but were loath to get involved, because they too were being bullied by Professor Sour. It seemed to all of us that nothing could be done to stop her abusive ways. We all learned to keep our heads down, to stay under the radar, and to look forward to graduation, when we would be rid of her. None of us considered confronting Professor Sour, nor did we believe that reporting her would prove helpful. So, on we went, being tormented by a bully and feeling powerless to do little else. And just when change looked impossible, something magical happened.

One evening, after a particularly challenging day with Professor Sour, I was sitting alone studying in the cafeteria when I was approached by another member of the nursing faculty (I'll call her Professor Sweet). I had only a couple of classes with Professor Sweet, but she was always friendly, well-prepared, and intelligent. She asked if she could join me, and I said, "Of course." After a bit of small talk, she asked me how I was doing. She seemed genuinely interested, but I learned long ago to keep my thoughts to myself and to avoid rocking the boat—especially where Professor Sour was concerned. So, I made some lame comment like, "I'm fine." But that response did not satisfy Professor Sweet. She sat patiently, probing me with her intelligent eyes, softly explaining that it was safe for me to speak candidly and from the heart. She urged me to take my time and assured me that I could trust her. I promised that I would give her offer serious thought.

Days later, I mustered the courage to approach Professor Sweet. She was earnest in her attempts to help me. Names and details remained unspoken, and we never spoke specifically about Professor Sour. Instead, we shared our mutual love for nursing and my hopes and dreams for the future. In her gentle, persuasive way, Professor Sweet helped rebuild my fractured self-esteem and restored my confidence. She encouraged me to stay in school, to pursue my dream of becoming a nurse, and to become a leader for nursing reform. I hung onto her every word. She mentored me and cultivated a love for nursing that had nearly been destroyed by Professor Sour. As I grew stronger under the healing guidance of Professor Sweet, I realized I had other allies around me. I reached out to them as well. Slowly, I began to trust again and to heal from the torment heaped upon me by Professor Sour. Ultimately, I believe with all my being that I am a nurse today because of the caring support of Professor Sweet and others like her. The experiences that happened to me so many years ago have largely defined my character and have influenced the nurse (and the person) I am today.

TELL-TALE SIGNS THAT YOU MIGHT BE THE TARGET OF INCIVILITY

You feel physically sick or emotionally upset before going to work or school.

You are the target of rude remarks, insults, or put-downs.

You are belittled, humiliated, or demeaned (often in front of others).

You are excluded, isolated, or marginalized from work, school, or social activities.

You are the object of teasing or practical jokes.

You are the target of gossip, rumors, or other types of offensive speech or behavior.

You are unreasonably overloaded with work or seemingly impossible deadlines (often without adequate resources to complete your responsibilities).

You are deliberately denied information or resources to be successful at work or school.

Coworkers intentionally withhold important information needed to perform well in your job.

You have been unsupported by a coworker and set up to fail.

You have been intentionally neglected, marginalized, or excluded by a coworker.

Confidences that you have shared with coworkers have been breached or shared without your permission.

As you read my story, which character resonated most with you? Was it the vulnerable young nursing student whose dreams for the future were nearly destroyed, yet who triumphed and succeeded in the end? Was it Professor Sour, whose atrocious behavior nearly ended an aspiring nursing career before it could even take flight? Or was it the empathetic bystanders who expressed understanding, but who also stayed silent out of fear and apprehension? Maybe it was Professor Sweet, whose kindness, courage, and caring audacity elevated me? Or possibly you can relate in some way to all four characters. Each of us has been vulnerable, and each of us has looked on without involving ourselves in adversity.

Moving From the Streets to the Academy

Though my story as a young nursing student is a compelling one—and one to which many of us can relate—it was only part of the impetus that influenced my quest for civility. I originally wrote about the following experience in *Reflections on Nursing Leadership* (Clark, 2012a). Before I started teaching in the university, I worked for more than a dozen years as a psychiatric nurse specializing in adolescent and family mental health issues. I was a member of a hotshot crew of adolescent mental health workers who treated a variety of mental health conditions and substance abuse disorders. Many of our patients were gang members, adjudicated youth with a history of violence. We used a primary prevention approach to help teenagers settle disputes and disagreements using words and other nonviolent means instead of using weapons and physical violence. We also considered protective factors and resilience measures to equip our patients with effective ways to deal with stress and to recover from traumatic life events, including trauma resulting from violence. My clinical work with aggressive and violent youth has fully informed my program of research on preventing organizational violence and continues to fuel my passion for creating civility, not only on college campuses but everywhere.

After leaving my clinical practice and taking a position as a university professor, in the beginning, things were fairly status quo. However, in the early 2000s, I began to witness attitudinal and behavioral changes in our nursing students. Some of the changes were subtle, but they set off alarm bells in my gut, because they reminded me of my earlier experiences with angry youth. Though my college students were not outwardly hostile, I noticed more and more rude and disruptive behaviors, and I wondered if it was "just me." I also wondered if my observations were even accurate—perhaps they were colored somewhat by my previous clinical work.

Armed with a probing and curious mind, I began my quest to learn all I could about this troubling phenomenon. I started asking other professors—much like a "man or woman-on-the-street" interview. I engaged in some of the most provocative conversations, and what I discovered was fascinating. Several professors were witnessing the same types of disruptive student behaviors, such as students consistently coming to class late, holding distracting side conversations, misusing cellphones, challenging faculty knowledge and credibility, and making harassing comments. Some professors told me they were retiring or moving on to other employment opportunities because of the toxic classroom behavior and the uncivil encounters that were psychologically and physically impacting their lives.

About the same time, two major events happened that forever changed my life and set the course for my program of study on incivility. One event involved a very angry nursing student who had failed a nursing course and, for some reason, held me responsible for the failure. Another faculty member had issued the failing grade, but because I was the course coordinator, I had to make the final decision about the grading outcome. I upheld the failure, but the student grieved the grade. Over the course of the student's attempts to "appeal" the failing grade, he made personal threats that to this very day make my heart race; in his anger and rage, he said things like, "You need to change this grade to a passing grade, because I know where you live, I know where you park your car, and I know where your kids go to school." It was a terrifying experience, and in retrospect, after a decade has passed, I see how far we have come in being able to deal with these situations and to prevent them from happening in the first place. Fortunately, this situation was safely resolved, but it left me a bit shell-shocked and questioning my desire to stay in my faculty role.

The second event happened about the same time and was much more chilling. It involved the killing of three university nursing professors, two of whom were shot in cold blood in a large lecture hall while students were taking their midterm exam. A third nursing professor was later found dead in her office. The shooter was a disturbed nursing student apparently enraged over being barred from the exam; he later turned the gun on himself and took his own life. Prior to the killings, the shooter mailed a lengthy manifesto to an area newspaper, detailing his plan to pull the trigger.

I knew then that I was onto something. I began to study this very important issue in earnest. My intrigue extended beyond student behaviors and grew to include faculty incivility and our potential contributions to the problem. My work includes student perceptions of the problem and garners their opinions about what can be done to effectively prevent, measure, address, and intervene in uncivil situations and what mobilizes us to resolve these issues. Over the years, my work has expanded to include the impact of incivility on patient safety in the practice environment and how nursing education and practice-based nurses can effectively collaborate to prepare both newly graduated and seasoned nurses to foster civil, healthy work environments.

Incivility is an issue that to some extent all of us face in American society. We are affected by these behaviors, whether it is road rage, desk rage, or just plain rudeness. Incivility is a damaging affront to human dignity and an assault on a person's intrinsic sense of self-worth. The effects can be devastating and long-lasting. Exposure to uncivil behaviors can result in physical symptoms, such as headaches, interrupted sleep, and intestinal problems, and can cause psychological conditions, including stress, anxiety, irritability, and depressive symptoms. Thus, we need to foster civility and to raise awareness about the importance of developing a civil and healthy academic and practice work environment.

Sometimes people say things like, "You know, Cindy, in our organization, incivility isn't really a problem, because only one or two individuals are uncivil or bully others." And here's my response: "Imagine you are a patient sitting with your primary care provider after undergoing a series of tests, and he or she says to you, 'No worries. Your tests and lab results are in. And, you are one of the lucky ones—you only have one or two malignant cells circulating throughout your body.'"

Yes, of course, this is a ridiculous (and insulting) response, but I suggest to you that the same level of ridiculousness relates to incivility in the work environment. It is my fervent belief, and the evidence bears this out, that one or two toxic employees (or students or faculty) can devastate an organization. For example, Porath and Pearson (2013) report that managers and executives of Fortune 1000 firms spend as much as 13% of their total work—or 7 full weeks per year—addressing problematic employee relationships or replacing workers who leave the organization because of incivility. In an earlier study, Pearson and Porath (2009) cite one example where a hospital spent more than $25,000 dealing with just one uncivil episode.

The costs of incivility are vast. Uncivil behavior adds to employer and employee stress levels, erodes self-esteem, damages relationships, and threatens workplace safety and quality of life (Forni, 2008). Incivility also lowers morale, causes illness, and leaves workers feeling stressed, vulnerable, and devalued. Therefore, creating and sustaining communities of civility is an imperative for all work environments as well as my life's work. My primary thesis is this: If we identify and address lesser acts of incivility before they escalate into aggression or violence, we are far better off, and in the end, the quality of life on all levels will be improved. And here's what I believe to my very core—civility *does* matter, and it is worth fighting the good fight to create and sustain healthy academic and practice workplaces where respect is highly regarded and where benevolence carries the day.

What Is Civility, and Why Does It Matter?

Several years ago, my colleague and I conducted a concept analysis of civility (Clark & Carnosso, 2008). We gathered information and readings from multiple disciplines, including political science, religion, philosophy, education, sociology, anthropology, and (to a lesser extent) nursing and other health sciences. We found that Sistare (2004) believes that civility requires tolerating, listening, and discussing differing viewpoints without acrimony, violence, or personal attacks. Similarly, Guinness (2008) defines civility as having respect for differences, discussing them robustly, and treating one another with dignity and honor. Emry and Holmes (2005) define civility as respect for others while honoring differences and seeking common ground. In our analysis, we distilled an abundance of information and thoughts on civility to ultimately construct an operational definition. Our concept analysis revealed that civility requires an authentic respect for the people involved and that each encounter requires time, presence, engagement, and intention to seek common ground.

On the surface, engaging in a civil conversation seems like an easy task. But in today's busy and rushed world, we are constantly bombarded with text and instant messaging, email, cellphone communication, and the use of other devices and social media that interrupt our daily activities and reduce the face time we used to enjoy with one another. If we are to be civil with one another, we each need to make time for intentional and purposeful dialogue. The goal should be to negotiate a mutual outcome, to avoid focusing on who's right and, instead, to find a common purpose and to agree to conduct ourselves in a civil and respectful manner.

What Is Incivility?

If *civility* is defined as the intention to seek common ground and inherently requires an authentic degree of respect for one another and the relationship, then what is incivility? Emry and Holmes (2005) define *incivility* as disregard and insolence for others, causing an atmosphere of disrespect, conflict, and stress. Overall, incivility is an assault on our human dignity and an injurious affront on our self-respect.

As we unwrap the layers of incivility, we discover that academic incivility may be defined as rude or discourteous speech or behavior that disrupts the academic environment (Feldman, 2001). Yet, this definition calls into question how one defines the "academic environment." Several years ago, I defined the academic environment as any location associated with the delivery of education, including the live or virtual classroom as well as the clinical setting (Clark, 2006). Since then, I have amended this definition to include "anywhere that teaching and learning occur." In other words, the academic environment can also include the campus square, nursing lounge, hallways and offices, or virtually anywhere there is a "teachable moment" for a conversation about civility to occur.

After we define the academic environment, we then consider the various dimensions of academic incivility. For example, student incivility toward faculty can be defined as rude or disruptive behavior that negatively impacts faculty levels of well-being, sense of self-worth, and commitment to teaching. Luparell (2004) measured nursing faculty's perception of student incivility in nursing education and found that some faculty described aggressive and severe incidents of student incivility. Most faculty members reported being verbally abused by students, and the effects of these encounters left negative and lasting impressions.

When I studied faculty incivility toward students, I discovered that students had a very similar experience. Students described faculty incivility as behavior that damages their confidence, erodes their sense of self-worth, and diminishes their psychological and physical well-being. I also found that student incivility toward faculty can have similar results (Clark, 2008a, 2008b).

Kathleen Heinrich (2006a, 2006b, 2007) has collected hundreds of stories from faculty in nursing education, asking participants to describe uncivil encounters with students, colleagues, and administrators. Heinrich coined the term *joy stealing* to describe nurse educators' conflicted relationships with student, colleague, and administrator *targets* that cause stress and drain zest in the work environment. She describes how the envy of excellence in academia by way of joy-stealing games "extinguish[es] zestful partnerships and hinders the pursuit of knowledge and scholarship" (Heinrich, 2006a, para. 34). The games described by Heinrich encompass 10 categorical destructive behaviors that feed feelings of disrespect, devaluing, or dismissal among faculty.

In 2013, I conducted a national study on faculty incivility which included nearly 600 respondents from more than 40 states in the United States (Clark, 2013; Clark, Olender, Kenski, & Cardoni, 2013). This mixed-methods study described experiences of incivility among and between nursing faculty, including academic nurse leaders. In this study, nearly 70% of the respondents perceived faculty incivility to be a moderate to serious problem. The respondents identified eight major types of behavior related to faculty incivility (see sidebar).

1. **Berating, insulting, and allowing:** *Verbal and nonverbal behaviors where respondents are insulted and/or berated; in many cases, these behaviors are tolerated and/or allowed to continue.*

2. **Setting up, undermining, and subverting:** *Coworkers deliberately sabotage, undermine, or set up colleagues to fail. In some cases, students are mobilized to undermine a faculty member.*

3. **Power playing, derailing, disgracing:** *Faculty inappropriately assert their position and often use others to "gang up on" (join forces against) another faculty member. These behaviors often include treating junior, adjunct, new, or clinical faculty, or faculty without the "right" degree, with disdain and disrespect.*

4. **Excluding, gossiping, and degrading:** *Faculty ignore, marginalize, shun, avoid, and exclude others. These behaviors also include conducting clandestine and secretive meetings, gossiping and spreading rumors, or degrading others by making age-related, racial, ethnic, gender, or religious slurs.*

5. **Refusing, not doing, and justifying:** *Faculty are not doing or refuse to do their share of the workload, or are being assigned an inequitable workload. Many faculty justify their lack of workload contributions by stating they have other urgent responsibilities and have more pressing or more important work to do.*

6. **Blaming and accusing:** *Faculty are blamed and falsely accused of something they did not do, often with no evidence of wrongdoing. Many times the accusations are ill-founded, but taken as truth nonetheless. The accused feel powerless to "prove" their innocence.*

7. **Taking credit for (ripping off) others' work:** *Sometimes subtle or blatant attempts at stealing and using a colleague's intellectual property and course content for their own gain or without obtaining permission or giving credit.*

8. **Distracting and disrupting during meetings:** *Faculty use computers or mobile devices, and/or engage in other non-meeting related activities (e.g., grading papers, having side conversations) during meetings.*

Incivility in nursing education is a moderate-to-serious problem (Clark et al., 2013; Clark & Springer, 2007a), and in my experience, whether the incivility occurs student to student, faculty to student, student to faculty, faculty to faculty, or in any other arrangement, the effects of the uncivil encounters often result in the "dance of incivility." The "dance" is an interactive, give-and-take process in which all participants are affected, and, ultimately, each person involved is responsible for creating a civil environment. The metaphor of a "dance" illustrates the reciprocity and interrelationship that might exist among faculty, students, staff, and administrators when incivility occurs.

For nearly 15 years, I have been exploring the serious nature of incivility and its potential consequences and conducting research and evidence-based studies to measure, prevent, minimize, and address incivility. As a result of these studies and after reading the work of other "civility scholars," I developed the following definition of incivility:

> *A range of rude or disruptive behaviors or failing to take action when action is warranted; these behaviors and inactions may result in psychological or physiological distress for the people involved—and if left unaddressed, may progress into threatening situations (or result in temporary or permanent illness or injury).* (Clark, 2009; Clark, C.M. & Kenski, D., 2017).

This definition has essentially four parts. The first and the fourth parts are consistent with the work of other authors.

The first part of the definition suggests that incivility includes rude or disruptive behaviors, and the fourth part focuses on our need to prevent minor encounters from escalating into more threatening situations, possibly resulting in temporary or permanent illness or injury.

It is the second and third parts of this definition to which I call your attention. First, the second part of the definition includes failing to take action when action is warranted; this part of the definition underscores the importance of how people can get hurt when we fail to speak up when uncivil encounters occur. The third part of the definition includes an emphasis on the psychological or physiological distress that might result from uncivil encounters. This is an exceedingly important issue. For well over a decade, I have been gathering stories from students, faculty, nurses in practice, other healthcare professionals, and nurse leaders in education and practice settings. Whether I gather the stories through face-to-face interviews or through written narratives, the impact of the uncivil encounter is frequently described as devastating and long-lasting. In fact, as people relate their stories, the experience seems so fresh that it is impossible for me to know when the uncivil encounter occurred unless the person tells me. The impact can often feel as though the encounter happened yesterday or in the very recent past, even though it might have happened 30 years ago. Individuals describe the effect of incivility as a powerful blow as they recount the psychological and physiological impact of the encounters. Some describe cardiac problems, migraine headaches, interrupted sleep, or gastric distress. Others describe the psychological trauma of incivility, including stress, anxiety, irritability, and depressive symptoms. In some cases, targets of incivility have been diagnosed with post-traumatic stress disorder and other serious mental and physical health disorders.

Uncivil behavior exists along a continuum ranging from disruptive behaviors on one end to threatening and violent behaviors on the other (see Figure 1.1; Clark, Barbosa-Leiker, Gill, & Nguyen, 2015).

These behaviors might be intentional or unintentional. By *unintentional,* I mean that in some cases, people exhibiting uncivil behaviors might be unaware of the effect of their behavior, words, or actions on others. The *Continuum of Incivility* illustrates that behaviors at the left end of the scale can be expressed by some fairly subtle behaviors, such as eye-rolling, arm-crossing, and walking away, and might progress to more overt expressions of incivility, such as bullying, taunting, and intimidation.

Continuum of Incivility

Clark © 2009, revised 2013, 2015
Latest Source: Clark, C. M., Barbosa-Leiker, C., Gill, L., & Nguyen, D. T. (2015). Revision and psychometric testing of the Incivility in Nursing Education (INE) Survey: Introducing the INE-R. *Journal of Nursing Education, 54*(6), 306–315.

FIGURE 1.1

Continuum of Incivility.

Whether intentional or unintentional, or low risk or high risk, uncivil behaviors can have harmful and lasting effects. For example, you might consider eye-rolling (on the far left of the continuum) an innocuous behavior; however, in my experience, eye-rolling can have negative and troubling effects. In my workshops I ask attendees, "Please raise your hand if others have rolled their eyes at you." In virtually every case, every hand is raised.

Then I ask, "How does it feel to have eyes rolled at you?" Their responses are forceful and compelling. Many comment that it makes them feel diminished, demeaned, unimportant, and angry, whereas others say they wish they could physically retaliate, though they do not, of course.

I then follow with another question—"What do you do about it?" The most common response is "nothing" and avoidance of the eye-roller; also, they stop asking questions. The problem is that not only do they stop asking questions of the eye-rolling offender, but also in many cases they stop asking questions altogether. This is a distressing outcome with far-reaching consequences. When nurses stop asking questions, patient care suffers. Even the most mundane, nonverbal uncivil behaviors, such as eye-rolling, can have serious consequences. Further, if eye-rolling can result in feelings of anger and avoidant behaviors, then what might be the effect of more disruptive and high-risk behaviors? What might be the short- and long-term impact of racial and ethnic slurs against our colleagues? How does an ongoing pattern of bullying affect the physiological and psychological well-being of our coworkers?

Finishing Touches

Acting civilly and respectfully is not always easy, especially in a high-stress learning environment, where constant change is the norm and where faculty and students experience complex and demanding workloads. Yet, we must make civility a priority for our students, colleagues, practice partners, and ourselves. Incivility takes a tremendous toll on everyone throughout the campus and practice community. Choosing civility is important and the right thing to do.

Some believe that pursuing civility is simply a fad that will hopefully pass quickly, while others believe that "civility" is just one more thing to add to their already full plate. I ascribe to the adage put forth by Dr. Vincent (2006, p. 28), who quipped, "Civility is not another piece to be added onto the plate of an educator, it 'is' the plate upon which all else is placed." I agree, and I am firmly convinced that civility is not only a choice but an important topic that must be addressed openly, deliberately, and explicitly.

CIVILITY TIP

Surround yourself with positive people. Seek and savor your "sweet spot" of civility—and then pay it forward. Become a supportive and encouraging mentor, coach, or friend to someone else. In time, and with a little bit of luck, the roots of civility will spread and deepen beyond your imaginings.

Chapter 2
The Costs and Consequences of Incivility: Rationale for Change

Civility costs nothing and buys everything. –Mary Wortley Montagu

This chapter discusses:

- The human and fiscal costs of incivility
- Reasons for addressing incivility
- Civility, ethical practice, and advancing our nation's health

The High Cost of Incivility

The costs of incivility are vast and impact us in myriad ways. Disruptive and intimidating behaviors can have negative and lasting effects on individuals, teams, and organizations. Years ago, I was deeply moved while reading the foreword of an excellent book authored by Pearson and Porath (2009), *The Cost of Bad Behavior: How Incivility Is Damaging Your Business and What to Do About It*. The foreword is written by Warren Bennis, a scholarly giant and consultant in the field of organizational leadership. Bennis titles the foreword "Little Murders" and writes a gripping account of his observations of incivility in the workplace in the late 1950s while studying doctor-nurse relationships. The story takes place in an operating-room theater between a gifted surgeon and an OR nurse. During a particularly grueling and lengthy surgical procedure, the surgeon grew more and more infuriated and demanding of the nurse. In his estimation, the nurse was too slow and failed to hand him the surgical instruments in a proper way. The surgeon screamed at the nurse in a profane and extremely demeaning manner. The nurse responded with her own level of rage by slamming the instruments into the surgeon's hand with such violent force that the doctor's palm was raw and reddened. Bennis and his colleagues later described the nurse's behavior as "spiteful obedience" and concluded that incivility is a pervasive condition in workplaces around the world, one that tends to be heightened when the world is suffering from discontent and uncertainty.

Bennis's graphic and vivid description of doctor-nurse incivility made a lasting impression on me. First, Bennis chose to focus on the business of healthcare to illustrate the costs and impact of incivility. For me, this was a jarring aspect of the story, because it was a story about us—the doctors and nurses whose job it is to deliver quality patient care and to advocate for patient safety. Second, to this day, I wonder what happened to the patient. What was the impact of such a fierce and aggressive encounter on the patient? I was left reeling from the account and was reminded once again about the serious consequences of incivility, particularly in healthcare, where the stakes are high and the outcome can result in life or death.

Porath and Pearson (2013) found that 98% of American workers reported experiencing incivility from coworkers and concluded that incivility occurs in "nearly all settings, by people of all ages, as part of their daily routine" (Pearson & Porath, 2009, p. 23). As a result, many workers are actively disengaged and less productive, and some intentionally undermine their organization and their coworkers. The authors present a set of action steps and mathematical equations to calculate the cost of even one uncivil employee in an organization. As an example, the authors describe the impact of one uncivil employee in a hospital—the costs of incivility escalate when one includes the expenses associated with supervising the employee, managing the situation, consulting with attorneys, and interviewing witnesses (doctors, nurses, patients, and others impacted by the offender or who witnessed the incivility). In this case, the hospital lost more than $25,000 as a result of one uncivil episode.

THE COSTS OF INCIVILITY AND ABUSIVE CONDUCT

27% of workers in the United States have experienced abusive conduct (bullying) at work.

37 million U.S. workers report being subjected to abusive conduct/bullying.

65.6 million workers are affected by abusive conduct/bullying (those abused + those who witness it).

72% of bullies are bosses.

58% of the targets are women.

80% of the time, female bullies target other women.

30% of bullied employees will resign from their jobs, and 20% of those who witness bullying will also leave the organization.

62% of employers ignore the problem.

45% of bullying targets suffer stress-related health problems.

40% of bullied individuals never tell their employers.

Only 3% of bullied people file lawsuits.

The annual cost to U.S. organizations is around $300 billion.

Pearson & Porath, 2009; Porath & Pearson, 2013; The Workplace Bullying Institute, 2014

This important information should be of interest to all employers and employees. As I mentioned in Chapter 1, I often hear people say, "We don't really have an incivility problem, because we only have one or two toxic employees, or just a few students who behave badly, or only a couple of uncivil faculty in our nursing school—so it's no big deal."

Again, I strongly contend that the cost of even one uncivil individual can have a deeply systemic effect and potentially devastate a workplace, and the evidence shows this contention to be true.

Clearly, incivility in the workplace is a serious problem. More than a decade ago, Farkas and Johnson (2002) found that 79% of survey respondents agreed that rudeness and incivility were growing and serious problems in the United States. In a more recent study by Weber Shandwick and Powell Tate (2013), investigators found that 70% of respondents believe that incivility in the United States has reached crisis levels, and 81% believe that uncivil behavior is leading to an increase in violence. In the same report, 37% of respondents personally experienced workplace incivility, 33% believed the general tone of the workplace is uncivil, and 26% have quit a job because it was an uncivil workplace. In the *Civility in America 2014* report (Weber Shandwick & Powell Tate, 2014), more than 9 in 10 of each adult generation believe that civility is a problem, and that incivility has reached crisis proportions in America. While it may be obvious that targets of incivility are harmed, Houshmand, O'Reilly, Robinson, and Wolff (2012) found that those who witnessed bullying in their workplace were more likely to resign, even though they themselves were not the target.

The academic setting is no exception. Clark and Springer (2010) studied academic nurse leaders' perceptions of incivility and found that student and faculty stressors, such as heavy work demands, financial pressures, and lack of administrative support, can lead to incivility. The academic nurse leaders in the study made several suggestions to address incivility and create cultures of civility in nursing education, including:

- Role-modeling civil, professional behavior
- Teaching and modeling direct, effective communication by seizing opportunities for engagement
- Creating cultures of mutual respect and emotional safety
- Encouraging freedom of expression and open, honest communication

Leaders need to initiate important conversations about civility by providing forums for open discussion and being visible and available to faculty and students. Additionally, academic nurse leaders play a key role in crafting vision statements and co-creating norms that reflect an emphasis on civility and respect. Olender-Russo (2009) suggested that the desired way the organization's members will treat themselves, each other, and the organization should be embedded within the organization's strategic plan, vision, mission, and values to increase the likelihood that change will occur and be sustained.

EXAMPLES OF MISSION STATEMENT, STATEMENT OF CIVILITY, AND SHARED VALUES

Mission: The University strives to create a campus culture that values civility, ethical behavior, professionalism, respectful discourse, and affirms the contributions of each member of the campus community.

Statement of Civility: All members of the University are dedicated to creating and maintaining a civil community that supports respectful discourse, openness to opposing points of view, and passionate argument. The display of ethical conduct and treating one another with respect is requisite to constructive communication and community building. Without civility, we miss opportunities to understand others' points of view and to find common ground. Civility is not equivalent to censorship, but instead is needed to bring decorum to discourse. This Statement of Civility is predicated on our shared values.

Shared Values:
  Academic excellence
  Respect
  Professionalism
  Ethical conduct
  Integrity and accountability
  Social justice
  Global citizenship

Source: Clark, in press.

In healthcare, academic, and other organizations, uncivil and disruptive behaviors might become embedded in the organizational culture and have a direct impact on employees as well as students and patients served by the organization. Incivility results in increased employee turnover, disruption of work teams, poor productivity, and significant economic loss (Pearson & Porath, 2009; Porath & Pearson, 2013; Weber Shandwick & Powell Tate, 2013, 2014). The stakes are even higher in healthcare settings where uncivil encounters can result in serious mistakes, preventable complications, and harm to or even death of a patient. Uncivil actions have detrimental effects on the health, well-being, and job satisfaction of nurses (Spence-Laschinger, Wong, Cummings, & Grau, 2014; Vessey, DeMarco, Gaffney, & Budin, 2009) and creates a heavy financial burden for healthcare organizations (Lewis & Malecha, 2011). The costs of incivility increase when expenses associated with supervising the employee, managing the situation, consulting with attorneys, and interviewing witnesses are considered (Griffin & Clark, 2014; Pearson & Porath, 2009; Porath & Pearson, 2013). The psychological impact of incivility on faculty and students may be devastating as well (Clark, 2008a, 2008b).

Creating a Culture of Safety: High Reliability Organizations (HROs) and Interprofessional Collaboration

A *high reliability organization* (HRO) is an organization that carries out complex, high-stakes work where mistakes can result in great harm. Weick and Sutcliffe (2007) define HROs as high-risk, dynamic, and potentially hazardous, while operating nearly error-free. Examples of HROs include amusement parks, the airline industry, nuclear power plants, and acute care hospitals. High reliability is not a new concept; however, as the healthcare industry moves from a fee-for-service model to one that is more consumer-driven, greater emphasis is placed on creating a culture of safety.

Focusing on a culture of safety is a healthcare imperative for all healthcare workers, including nurses. In 2016, the American Nurses Association named "A Culture of Safety" as its annual theme. Becoming an HRO is an important way to address this decree, and more and more healthcare organizations are striving to achieve this designation. According to Oster & Braaten (2016), three key elements are necessary to become an HRO: leadership commitment, investment in a culture of safety, and the use of continuous quality improvement processes to ultimately improve the systems of healthcare delivery and foster safe working environments. To create a culture of safety, the authors challenge nurses (and other healthcare workers) to consistently ask the following questions (p. xxviii):

1. Is this the most current practice?

2. Is this the safest way to do this (practice/treatment/procedure)?

3. What are possible "errors waiting to happen" that we can prevent?

HROs have systems in place that make them exceptionally consistent in accomplishing their goals and avoiding potentially catastrophic errors. There is an intentional commitment to safety at all levels—from all workers, providers, managers, and administrators.

Fostering a culture of safety in healthcare includes a commitment to creating and sustaining positive work environments by promoting civility, professionalism, and ethical practice. Building a culture of safety includes investing in the 200% rule (Maxfield, Grenny, Lavendro, & Groah, 2011), which goes like this: Each member of the healthcare team is 100% responsible for his or her own individual commitment to patient safety, and 100% responsible for making sure that all other members of the healthcare team are focused on patient safety as well. This commitment can be verbal or written. In a critical access hospital in Idaho, all members of the healthcare team have committed the 200% rule in writing, and have posted the signed document to make it more official and a part of the everyday work experience. Thankfully, the days of working in silos are over, and the era of functioning as a valued member of a multi-disciplined, multi-talented, high-performing team is happily here to stay. In today's healthcare environment, nurses are integral and valued members of a multi-skilled, interprofessional team of workers representing a variety of professional backgrounds working together with patients, families, and communities to deliver the highest quality of care. The Interprofessional Education Collaborative Expert Panel (2011) developed four domains for interprofessional collaborative practice:

1. **Values/Ethics:** Showing mutual respect and ascribing to shared values

2. **Roles/Responsibilities:** Understanding and valuing the roles and responsibilities of other healthcare professions

3. **Interprofessional Communication:** Using communication that supports a team approach and patient-centered care

4. **Teams and Teamwork:** Focusing on relationship building, shared values, and common principles

High-functioning teams play an integral role in fostering civil, healthy work environments. By now it should be crystal clear: Incivility in the healthcare setting can have a devastating and long-lasting effect on individuals, teams, organizations, and patient care. As nurse educators, we have an unequivocal responsibility to conduct ourselves in an ethical manner consistent with our codes of ethics and other professional statements.

Civility, Ethics, and Advancing Our Nation's Health

No matter where we practice, regardless of position, setting, specialty, or status, all nurses have an ethical obligation to create and sustain healthy workplaces and to foster an atmosphere of dignity and respect. Every year since 1999 (except 2001 following the 9/11 attacks, when first responders were rated higher), Americans responding to Gallup polls rated nurses highest on honesty and ethical standards (Gallup, 2016). While this distinction is impressive, nurses need to earn this high honor. Paying close attention to how we conduct ourselves both privately and professionally speaks to our character and our moral make-up.

Nursing practice is guided by codes of ethics outlining ethical conduct and responsibilities for all nurses. The International Council of Nurses (ICN) *Code of Ethics for Nurses* (ICN, 2012) emphasizes the nurse's responsibility to respect human rights, treat others with dignity and respect, and provide respectful and unrestricted care. Additionally, the American Nurses Association (ANA) *Code of Ethics for Nurses with Interpretive Statements (The Code)* clearly articulates all nurses' obligation to foster safe, ethical, civil workplaces (ANA, 2015a). I'd like to highlight two specific provisions within *The Code* that speak directly to fostering civility and healthy work environments. The first example is a brilliant revision to *The Code* that made me jump for joy and extend high fives to anyone who'd join me in my exuberance. I *love* how emphasis is placed on civility and kindness—this is a perfect way to express nurses' obligation to foster healthy work environments. The second example speaks directly to the role nurse educators play in preparing students to foster healthy workplaces.

1. Provision 1.5 requires nurses "to create an ethical environment and culture of civility and kindness, treating colleagues, co-workers, employees, students, and others with dignity and respect...and that any form of bullying, harassment, intimidation, manipulation, threats or violence will not be tolerated" (p. 4).

2. Provision 7.2 requires academic educators to "ensure that all graduates possess the knowledge, skills, and moral dispositions that are essential to nursing" (p. X).

These codes of ethics support the requirement that nurses in all areas of nursing education and practice display civil behaviors continuously. The ANA's *Nursing: Scope and Standards of Practice* (2015c) also provides a framework of objective guidelines to promote accountability of nurses for their actions, including how they relate to patients and peers. In addition, the ANA standards of professional performance are clear standards and objective guidelines for nurses to be accountable for their actions, their patients, and their peers. In particular, the professional performance standard of ethics, quality of practice, communication, and collaboration is central to building and fostering communities and cultures of civility.

Several other organizations are helping point the way back to civility as they help advance the nation's healthcare system. In 2008, the Robert Wood Johnson Foundation (RWJF) and the Institute of Medicine (IOM) collaborated to assess and transform the nursing profession and to produce an action-oriented blueprint for the future of nursing. In 2011, the IOM report called for substantial transformation in nursing roles in all sectors of healthcare and for nursing education to take greater professional responsibility to prepare this new generation of nurse leaders. As the largest component of the healthcare population, nurses are uniquely positioned to lead change at all levels of the healthcare system—including creating healthy and civil workplaces in nursing education. To do so, nurses must increase their leadership capacity to implement transformational change, redefine the future, align people, and inspire action to achieve a compelling vision and realize meaningful results. Ultimately, the report centered on four key messages (IOM, 2011):

1. Nurses should practice to the full extent of their education and training.

2. Nurses should achieve higher levels of education and training through an improved education system that promotes seamless academic progression.

3. Nurses should be full partners, with physicians and other health professionals, in redesigning healthcare in the United States.

4. Effective workforce planning and policymaking require better data collection and information infrastructure.

In addition to these key messages, the IOM report issued eight specific recommendations. I would like to highlight three of the eight recommendations:

- **Recommendation 2:** Expand opportunities for nurses to lead and diffuse collaborative improvement efforts.

- **Recommendation 7:** Prepare and enable nurses to lead change to advance health.

- **Recommendation 8:** Build an infrastructure to collect and analyze healthcare workforce data.

I selected these three recommendations to provide rationale for fostering civility, because to some extent each requires doctors, nurses, and other healthcare professionals to work together and because they underscore the need for collaboration, teamwork, and collegiality—which are all highly related to establishing and sustaining respectful and civil interactions. None of these recommendations will be easy to accomplish. We must establish civil and respectful relationships and interactions to accomplish these important and necessary goals.

The American Association of Colleges of Nursing (AACN) *Essentials of Baccalaureate Education for Professional Nursing Practice* (2008) includes 11 essentials designed to transform baccalaureate nursing education by "providing the curricular elements and framework for building the baccalaureate nursing curriculum for the 21st century" (p. 4). Of these essentials, Essential VIII: Professionalism and Professional Values (and behaviors associated with this category) is foundational to the practice of nursing. Essential VIII underscores the importance of professionalism and the inherent understanding of the historical, legal, and contemporary context of nursing practice. Professionalism includes being accountable and taking responsibility for individual actions and behaviors, including civility. In other words, civility must be present for professionalism to occur.

Magnet® recognition in healthcare organizations conveys that an agency is an exceptional place to work, as evidenced by the delivery of excellent patient care, high levels of job satisfaction, low turnover rates, and collective decision-making among members of the healthcare team. Magnet facilities reflect positive, dynamic, and responsive organizational cultures guided by leaders who support participation, feedback, and communication (American Nurses Credentialing Center [ANCC], 2016; Dumpel, 2010). Achieving Magnet status in practice organizations is a pinnacle of achievement. The 14 Forces of Magnetism include the members' ability to work together and to collaborate to improve patient outcomes and healthcare delivery systems. This is another rationale for promoting civility. If civility is not present, it is unlikely that the Forces of Magnetism can be achieved and ultimately sustained. In some way, all of the 14 Forces of Magnetism require civility and respect; however, four of the forces stand out as being closely related to civility:

- **Force 3:** Management Style relies on a supportive, participative work environment where feedback is encouraged, valued, and incorporated at all levels of the organization.

- **Force 4:** Personnel Policies and Programs reflects safe and healthy work environments that provide opportunities for professional growth and that provide policies and programs to support professional nursing practice, work/life balance, and the delivery of quality care.

- **Force 6:** Quality of Care provides for a work environment that positively influences patient outcomes and where high-quality care to patients occurs.

- **Force 13:** Interdisciplinary Relationships emphasizes the value of collaborative working relationships within and among the various healthcare disciplines where mutual respect exists and where conflict management strategies are in place and are used effectively.

The Quality and Safety Education for Nurses (QSEN, 2016) competencies are designed to "prepare future nurses with the knowledge, skills, and attitudes (KSAs) necessary to continuously improve the quality and safety of the healthcare systems within which they work" (p. 1). The QSEN competencies are based on the IOM (2003) competencies. Though nearly all of them rely on civility and respect, the competencies of Patient Safety and Teamwork and Collaboration exemplify civility— these competencies call for functioning effectively within nursing and interprofessional teams and fostering open communication, mutual respect, and shared decision-making to achieve safe, quality patient care. More specifically, the Teamwork and Collaboration competency requires nurses to act with integrity and respect for differing views, to appreciate the importance of intra- and interprofessional collaboration, to respect the unique attributes of team members, to initiate actions to resolve conflict, and to use communication that minimizes risk to patient safety. All these skills and attitudes are reliant upon civil relationships and teamwork.

Regulatory Response—Game Over

Another strong rationale for fostering civility is The Joint Commission (TJC) sentinel event alert released in July 2008, with a go-live date of January 2009. In this alert, TJC noted that healthcare settings are high-stakes, pressure-packed environments that can test the limits of civility in the workplace—and that rude and disruptive behavior among healthcare professionals can pose a serious threat to patient safety and overall quality of care. TJC promulgated a new leadership standard (LD.03.01.01) to address intimidating, disruptive, and inappropriate behavior in accredited healthcare organizations. This sentinel alert addresses behavior that undermines a culture of safety, because it seriously threatens patient safety and employee satisfaction. According to TJC, uncivil, disruptive, and intimidating behavior in healthcare can lead to medical errors, poor patient care and satisfaction, preventable adverse patient outcomes, and increased costs of care. Incivility also causes qualified clinicians, administrators, and managers to seek new positions in more professional environments.

The leadership standard addresses a continuum of disruptive behavior that includes covert actions, such as withholding important information from others and failing to cooperate with colleagues, and overt actions, such as verbal threats and blatant acts of intimidation. Overt acts of intimidation and coercion constitute bullying and are clearly unacceptable.

Nurses, physicians, administrators, nonclinical staff, or other members of the organization might be instigators or targets of uncivil or bullying behavior. In some cases, this behavior becomes embedded in the organizational culture and has a direct impact on employees as well as patients entrusted to their care. As a result, TJC requires healthcare organizations to recognize and address behavior that threatens patient safety and the performance of the healthcare team. TJC recommended that all accredited healthcare organizations create behavioral codes of conduct and establish a formal process for managing unacceptable behaviors.

I like to call TJC's sentinel event alert the first of two significant and important bookends on the quest to create civil workplaces for healthcare workers. The second of the two bookends includes a regulatory response from some state boards of nursing (BON) that are beginning to sanction nursing programs for uncivil conduct among faculty and students. In one state, a nursing program was cited for incivility and required to develop a defined set of expectations, interventions, strategies, and written policies to improve the culture of academic civility. The program was also required to produce evidence of a respectful, confidential, positive, and productive academic environment and improved student-faculty relationships and communication to ensure student success. If this did not happen, the school of nursing might be closed. I was fortunate to be included in the intervention study that subsequently ensued (Clark, 2011).

In the summer of 2009, the director of the nursing program called me to explain that the program had been cited by the BON for faculty, student, and practice partner incivility. A number of faculty and students lodged complaints about the type and level of incivility occurring in the nursing program, and members of the practice community had expressed concern about the disrespectful and occasionally intimidating behavior displayed by some of the nursing faculty. Students felt victimized by faculty and complained about the use of scare tactics and bullying behaviors. Faculty-to-faculty incivility was another concern. The BON required the program to develop a clearly defined set of expectations, strategies, and written policies "to enhance student-faculty relationships and to improve the culture of academic civility." Further, the consequences of not taking action were dire. Significant improvements needed to be demonstrated within 6 months; otherwise, the program would be closed. Given the seriousness of the situation, the director requested my assistance to address the problem.

The team developed and implemented an ambitious and multi-dimensional intervention plan to include preintervention and postintervention institutional assessments, an evidence-based framework for establishing collaborative partnerships, and a series of day-long workshops with faculty and students. An action research approach provided a structure for collaboration and an effective method to organize our processes. The nursing director, faculty, and students were full members in the intervention plan. The institutional assessments provided scientific evidence to understand the type and frequency of faculty and student incivility and its effects on the learning environment and to develop practical strategies to address the problem. Using Heinrich's framework for establishing collaborative partnerships (Heinrich, 2010b; Heinrich, Clark, & Luparell, 2008) and conducting day-long faculty and student workshops were vital to the success of the plan. The workshops were carefully planned to include both structured and unstructured activities, and valuable time was spent in thoughtful conversation and problem-solving efforts to identify and practice individual and collective civility strategies. With few exceptions, each member of the faculty and student body implemented strategies to fulfill the vision to foster civility in the program. In the end, a well-planned intervention strategy helped align a dedicated group of faculty and students to take initial steps toward fulfilling their vision of civility and achieving lasting results. This beginning transformation serves as an example of the positive changes that can occur when faculty, students, and academic leaders come together to foster a culture of civility and change.

Finishing Touches

The costs and associated consequences of incivility are vast and troubling. And the toll it takes on individuals, teams, and organizations can be disturbing. Though civility matters for many important reasons, at the end of the day, it simply matters because it is the right thing to do. As a wise person once said, "If it were easy [in this case, behaving in a civil manner], everyone would do it." I realize that our days are often hectic, the workload sometimes seems unmanageable, and other days our patience is in short supply, yet patience is a virtue that makes all of us better. Seeking support and setting a positive example to lead the transformation for cultivating civility in nursing education are not easy but definitely worth the effort.

CIVILITY TIP
Become a catalyst and a change agent in your nursing program. Take the lead to rewrite the narrative on civility and how it can be embedded in your vision and mission statements and shared values and threaded through your everyday interactions with colleagues and students.

Chapter 3

The Inextricable Link Between Stress and Incivility

Students and faculty are under tremendous stress and do not always respect one another. When stress increases, the potential for conflict also increases, which in turn, increases the potential for incivility.
–Nurse educator

This chapter discusses:

- Putting incivility in context
- Understanding the relationship between stress and incivility
- Dealing with badly behaving people
- Choreographing the dance of civility

Incivility in Context

Incivility in nursing education does not exist in a vacuum; instead, it is a microcosm of the greater American society and, thus, must be situated in context. By just about any measure, incivility is on the rise, and goodwill and decorum are declining in our nation. Many Americans believe that incivility has worsened over the past several years and often cite our fast-paced society, high-tech information age, and increasing stress levels as major contributors to the problem.

In April 2016, the Associated Press-NORC Center for Public Affairs Research (2016) released the results of a survey revealing Americans' beliefs about civility in the United States. The survey was completed by more than 1,000 adult respondents and was particularly interesting because it was conducted during the presidential election year. Overall, the majority of respondents (74%) believe that civility has deteriorated in America over the past several decades. Further, many expressed their concern about incivility in American politics. In particular, the Republican campaign was viewed as rude and disrespectful (78%), nearly double the perception of the Democratic campaign (41%). The study further revealed that clear differences exist between younger and older Americans in terms of behaviors considered to be uncivil. For example, younger Americans believe that it is acceptable to use cellphones in restaurants and movie theaters, while only 22% of those over age 60 agree.

Similarly, findings from the *Civility in America 2016* report (Weber Shandwick & Powell Tate, 2016) found that civility continues to be a societal concern. Of the 1,005 survey respondents reporting, 95% believe that incivility is a problem, and 74% report that civility has declined over the past few years. Remarkably, 70% believed that incivility in America has risen to "crisis" levels, and in terms of politics, 93% report that a candidate's tone or level of civility matter and will be an important factor in deciding how they cast their votes in the 2016 presidential election. Regrettably, yet understandably, 64% say they have stopped paying attention to political conversations and debates because of the negative tone and only 38% accept the notion that incivility is just part of the political process.

Respondents identified politicians, the Internet/social media, and the news media as the top three sources contributing most to the lack of civility in American society. Interestingly, Americans view themselves as quite civil; 94% say they are always or usually polite and respectful, yet only 20% think the American people usually or always behave civilly. This is an illuminating finding; the disparity between how an individual views herself/himself versus the perception he or she has about others will be further discussed in Chapter 5.

In an earlier report, Weber Shandwick and Powell Tate (2014) found that 70% of respondents believe that incivility in the United States has reached crisis levels, and 81% believe that uncivil behavior is leading to an increase in violence. In the same report, 37% of respondents personally experienced workplace incivility, 33% believed the general tone of the workplace is uncivil, and 26% have quit a job because it was an uncivil workplace. The researchers contend that the more incivility infiltrates our culture and the more indifferent we become to its effects, the more likely we are to pass our tolerance of incivility to the next generation. As a result, the majority (65%) of respondents reported the need for broad-based civility training and called for a national public education campaign, including schools, cities, and public squares across America, to turn the tide on incivility.

Stress: A Crippling and Contributing Factor

For the past 8 years, the American Psychological Association (APA) has published a nationwide survey to examine the state of stress across the United States and to understand its impact. According to the APA, the Stress in America survey measures attitudes and perceptions of stress, leading sources of stress, common behaviors used to manage stress, and the impact of stress on American lives (APA, 2016). The results of the 2015 survey (released March 10, 2016) draw attention to the serious levels of stress caused by discrimination, the toll that stress takes on our personal health, and the serious lack of access to healthcare.

The 2015 survey included 3,361 American adults who identified several major stressors. Since 2007, stress related to money and work have topped the list. The 2015 survey showed similar results with money and work rated at 67% and 65%, respectively; however, for the first time, the 2015 survey found that family responsibilities were the third most common stressor (54%) followed by personal health concerns (51%), and health problems affecting their family (50%).

The 2015 survey also revealed that American adults experience extreme stress levels (24%), have at least one chronic illness (67%), and more than 10% report having a mental health–related diagnosis such as depression (16%) and anxiety disorders (13%). Physical illnesses are also a concern, with 32% of respondents reporting high blood pressure and 58% being overweight or obese. Many adults report being sedentary for much of the day (average of 6.4 hours per day) by sitting or lying without much movement, spending time at a desk, watching TV, or using a computer. Thirty-nine percent of adults report overeating or eating in other unhealthy ways due to stress, changes in sleeping habits (33%), headaches (32%), and an inability to concentrate (27%) due to stress.

Further, results revealed that stress affects behavior—almost half of adults who have a spouse or partner (47%) reported losing patience with or yelling at that spouse in the past month when they were feeling stressed. Twenty-five percent of the employed respondents reported snapping at or being short with coworkers because of stress.

Forni (2008) contends that nearly 1 million workers miss work every day because of workplace stress—a condition closely related to incivility. Rude behavior and other forms of incivility are damaging on multiple levels, including adding to workers' stress level, eroding self-esteem, damaging relationships, and threatening workplace safety and quality of life. Incivility lowers morale, causes illness, and leaves workers feeling stressed, vulnerable, and devalued. The human and financial costs of these behaviors can be disastrous and cannot be overstated.

Pearson and Porath (2009) also assert that stress associated with incivility costs businesses in myriad ways. Stress stemming from incivility, including the stress caused by ignoring incivility, can result in absenteeism, loss of productivity, and escalating healthcare costs. The authors contend that when organizations and leaders overlook incivility and associated stress factors, they ultimately risk losing valuable employees, because the more uncivil the work environment, the more stressed the employees, and the more likely they are to seek employment elsewhere. Stress and incivility also have a significant psychological and physical impact. Put simply, stress wreaks havoc on the workplace. Stress is associated with weight loss and gain, headaches, high blood pressure, and sleep disturbances. It also leads to loss of concentration, decreases productivity, and thwarts creativity. If an individual is exposed to incivility for too long or too often, significant health problems can occur, including cardiovascular disease, mental health disorders, autoimmune disorders, cancer, and diabetes. Stress impairs learning, work performance, and productivity. Workers might withdraw by neglecting their job responsibilities or think about exiting the organization. In the end, an uncivil work environment robs individuals of their self-respect and kills the human spirit.

Why Some People Behave Badly—Stress as a Major Contributor

I am often asked what motivates people to behave badly and engage in uncivil acts. This is not a simple question. In fact, for every negative or harmful act, there is a corresponding reason or explanation. Some of the explanations make sense, while others simply fail to explain the true nature of disrespectful human interactions. To address this provocative question, the following entry is excerpted from my *Musing of the Great Blue* blog posting (Clark, 2016):

First, do you consider yourself a reasonably respectful or civil person? Most of us would say yes. If this is true for you, here's another question: Have you ever been rude or disrespectful to someone? If you are like every other human being, the answer to the second question is also yes. So then the question becomes, why would an otherwise civil or respectful person behave rudely or badly? Very often, the answer is, "Because I'm stressed out." I agree; heightened levels of stress brought on by any number of life's demands often account for much incivility. Stress may be caused by the challenges of managing the myriad roles and responsibilities associated with family, work, and life in general. Being overworked, underpaid, and sometimes unappreciated also may contribute to increased stress. Although not acceptable, responding rudely in highly stressful situations is more easily understood than other forms of incivility.

In the workplace, incivility can add tension to an already highly stressed environment, and its potential impact cannot be overestimated. Being treated badly or in an uncivil manner, particularly over time, can have devastating results. In a practice-based discipline, such as nursing, this is especially troubling, because incivility can weaken confidence and moral courage; impair clinical judgment and reasoning; create vulnerability and self-doubt; and cause anxiety, resentment, and anger. Ultimately, it can negatively impact patient care.

Stress is not the only contributor to incivility. I'm reminded of a story told to me by a nursing instructor in her mid-50s. She was so excited because she had finally, after much soul-searching and research, decided to pursue a doctoral degree. She could hardly wait to share her excitement and ideas with her program director. When she had an opportunity to meet with the director and disclose her scholarly intentions, the director laughed and said, "Are you kidding, at your age? You can't be serious. By the time you finish your degree, you'll be ready to retire. We prefer to invest in younger faculty."

The exchange left the instructor feeling demoralized and diminished, and she decided to forgo pursuing the doctoral degree. Whether the director's comments were intentionally or unintentionally delivered, the result was the same: A talented and energetic faculty member was left to feel devalued and unimportant.

This example illustrates the negative impact that low emotional intelligence, ineffective communication skills, and an attitude of superiority—a sense of *power over*—can have. The instructor in this story is the target of rankism, a term coined by Robert W. Fuller, PhD, former president of Oberlin University. In his book, *Somebodies and Nobodies: Overcoming the Abuse of Rank*, Fuller tells us that "rankism" lies at the heart of discriminatory behavior, is evident in nearly every institution in society, and occurs when people abuse their power to demean and disadvantage those they outrank (2003).

Intended or not, disrespectful and rude behavior toward others may indicate prejudice and rise to the level of discrimination—in some cases, outright abuse. The antidote to rankism is to foster work environments based on human dignity for all. It is abuse of power and rank—not power and rank per se—that damages relationships and puts people at a disadvantage.

Those who are targets of rankism and other forms of incivility often describe their experiences in vividly emotional ways. Many are still negatively impacted by their uncivil experiences, even when the encounters occurred years before. Some people describe intense psychological symptoms, such as feeling traumatized, helpless, and powerless. Many feel caught in a no-win situation, with little possibility of successful resolution. The lingering effects of incivility can cause serious and sometimes lasting psychological and physiological effects.

Although each of us deserves to be treated with dignity and respect, people report varying degrees of discomfort when addressing conflict and incivility. For further discussion of this topic, refer to Chapter 8.

If you have been the target of repeated incivility or bullying, attending to your physical, emotional, and spiritual health is a critical first step. It may be necessary to see your healthcare provider or seek counsel from a mental-health expert. Getting yourself physically and emotionally prepared to deal with the problem will require you to be in a healthy state. When reporting a problem, it's important to follow confidentiality policies, procedures, and guidelines (assuming they exist). In any case, inform your employer or supervisor about the problem, and request institutional support. Be sure that human resource and employee-assistance program personnel have your best interests in mind and are poised to assist you in following healthy workplace policies and procedures.

If you experience incivility, either inside or outside the workplace, you need to reverse the negative effects it can have on your physical, emotional, and spiritual well-being. If you have been the target of bad behavior, here are 10 tips for successful recovery.

1. Share your story with a good friend, family member, mentor, counselor, or member of the clergy. Avoid sharing your experience with coworkers. Instead, seek support from those who can offer a more objective perspective, such as an ombudsperson, conflict negotiator, or civility coach. Relating the experience and sharing it with others can provide healing. However, avoid dwelling on it too long. Tell your story, validate that it occurred, and make a plan to move forward.

2. Journal about your experience. For many people, writing their story and reflecting on it can be therapeutic and may help provide insight.

3. Engage in activities you enjoy, and don't retreat from relationships that matter to you. Continue to make time for exercise, friends, family, pets, and social activities.

4. Enjoy a massage, meditation, yoga, deep breathing exercises, and other relaxation techniques.

5. Get plenty of sleep, stay hydrated, and eat a well-balanced diet.

6. Get (or stay) involved by helping a friend, neighbor, or co-worker. Volunteer in the community, or champion one of your favorite causes.

7. Focus on building resiliency. No one size fits all, so find the plan that works for you. Surround yourself with positive people and with those who bring you joy.

8. Try to find meaning in stressful or traumatic events and experiences, and incorporate this meaning into moving forward.

9. Recognize what makes you uniquely strong, and own it! Don't let others define you. Memorize and practice reciting a positive script, such as: "I am poised, balanced, and in control of my life. I am talented, courageous, and confident in my ability to succeed."

10. Remember, symptoms of distress can last from a few days to many months, and recovery takes time and progresses at varying paces and degrees. If symptoms are persistent, you may need to talk with an expert. Don't hesitate to reach out for support if you need it.

Dealing With Incivility in the Workplace

Failure to address incivility degrades the teaching-learning environment, impairs relationships, and may eventually harm the reputation of the school. In nursing and other health-related disciplines, the impact of incivility can extend well beyond the academic setting and negatively affect patient safety. In healthcare, the consequences of incivility can result in life-threatening mistakes, preventable complications, and harm or even death of a patient. As the body of science grows about the negative impact of incivility on academic and patient care environments, leaders from both settings are seeking solutions to address the problem. If you or someone you know is experiencing workplace incivility, in addition to the 10 tips for recovery, the strategies offered in the nearby sidebar may also be helpful.

DEALING WITH INCIVILITY IN THE WORKPLACE

Begin with yourself—take a personal inventory (assess your Clark Workplace Civility Index, as seen in Chapter 5).

Seek honest feedback about your Clark Workplace Civility Index with a trusted colleague.

Make your physical and mental health a priority.

Live your best life—as George Herbert reminds us, "Living well is the best revenge."

Stay civil, but detached: Do not feed into the negativity.

Reduce stress and engage in self-care activities.

Surround yourself with positive people.

Talk with a trusted friend or a counseling professional.

Avoid contact with uncivil colleague(s) as much as possible.

Work from home as much as your work responsibilities allow.

Schedule shorter meetings where the uncivil colleague is present.

Communicate with an uncivil colleague by telephone or email rather than in person.

Ask to be reassigned to teams or committees (if uncivil colleague is a member).

Avoid meeting with the uncivil colleague(s) alone.

Hone and practice your communication skills, be assertive, and address the offender.

Try not to personalize or take offense—the offender might enjoy getting a rise out of you.

Document the behaviors and use organizational guidelines to address the behavior.

Raise awareness and enlist help from organizational leaders (for example, Human Resources).

continues

Assess your commitment to the organization—explore other options and opportunities.

The detrimental impact of workplace incivility is well documented, and if allowed to take root, the consequences can be extreme. If you find yourself working in an unhealthy or toxic work environment, consider the toll it may be taking on your physical, mental, and spiritual well-being. It may be time to move on and seek an enjoyable workplace where you can truly thrive in your career and profession.

The Academy: The Last Citadel of Civility

Some consider institutions of higher education to be the last citadel of civility and the last bastion of decorum in our society. In the sentinel work *Campus Life: In Search of Community* (1990), the Carnegie Foundation for the Advancement of Teaching authors reinforced the need for members of the campus community to develop a civil society where colleges and universities are open communities, where freedom of expression is protected, and where civility is affirmed. Yet, to some extent, the academy is failing to create and sustain communities of civility. Stress is a contributing factor to this perceived failure. Each semester, the American College Health Association (ACHA) conducts the National College Health Assessment (NCHA)—a nationally recognized research survey about college students' health habits, behaviors, and perceptions. The NCHA provides timely and relevant data about student health by measuring the top factors that present a barrier to student academic performance. Year after year, stress is identified as a barrier to student academic performance and success. In fall 2015, 30% of students reported that stress affected their academic performance, 36% of students reported higher-than-average levels of stress, and 11% reported tremendous levels of stress (ACHA, 2015).

Our nation's college students also suffer from a variety of psychological and emotional issues, including anxiety and mood disorders, substance abuse and eating disorders, learning disabilities, and relationship problems (Arehart-Treichel, 2002; Kadison & DiGeronimo, 2004). Types of students susceptible to increased stress include adult re-entry students who might hold a previous degree in another field or have worked in another profession, students who want to earn a nursing degree in a depressed job market, and others who return to college to achieve their dream of becoming a nurse. Students are also faced with significant financial concerns related to soaring tuition costs, lack of student-loan programs, high gas prices, and costs associated with the stress from dealing with the competing demands of school, work, and family. My own work (Clark, 2008a, 2008b) reveals similar findings, such as burnout from juggling multiple roles, competing in a high-stakes academic environment, financial worries, and exposure to faculty and student conflict.

In a more recent report (Clark, Nguyen, & Barbosa-Leiker, 2014) we conducted a 3-year longitudinal study to measure a cohort of prelicensure nursing students' progressive perceptions of stress, coping, student-student and faculty-student relationships, and levels of academic civility. The top three stressors for nursing students remained consistent over the 3-year study period:

1. Demanding academic workloads

2. Balancing time, work, school, and family

3. Finding time to relax

Other stressors included financial concerns, grade competition, and sleep problems. As time in their nursing program progressed, students identified additional stressors not reported in the first year of the study including faculty incivility, stress related to studying for the licensing examination (NCLEX), achieving required scores on placement examinations, and fear of failure. The top three most effective coping strategies also remained consistent over the 3-year study period:

1. Talking and spending time with family, friends, and pets

2. Exercising and getting outdoors

3. Organizing, planning, and prioritizing

Other coping strategies included engaging in self-care activities and seeking help from supportive faculty and/or professional counselors.

While civility scores remained mild to moderately high overall, there was a slightly declining trend over the 3-year period. Interestingly, student relationships with faculty played a key role in maximizing perceptions of civility. Respondents suggested various ways to improve student-faculty relationships including using effective and timely communication, faculty encouragement, organization, and flexibility, engaging with faculty in social/extracurricular activities, providing open forums for a dialogue about civility, establishing and enforcing behavioral norms, and providing opportunities for stress-reducing activities.

In another study conducted with nearly 5,000 nursing students from all 50 United States and the District of Columbia enrolled in all program levels of nursing (Clark, 2014), I asked nursing students to identify their top three stressors. They included:

1. Curricular demands such as assignments, exams, group work, and clinical preparation

2. Time management (balancing work, school, family, personal relationships, and self-care)

3. Pressure to succeed accompanied by a fear of failure

Many students expressed worry that after all they had invested in completing their nursing program, they still may fail the licensing exam and/or be unable to find employment. In this same study, I also asked students to identify their top three coping strategies. These included:

1. Talking and spending time with family, friends, and pets

2. Participating in relaxation and self-care activities such as massage, watching TV, listening to music, cooking, reading, and meditating

3. Organizing, planning, and prioritizing their school, family, and work lives

Further, I asked students to rate their level of stress while enrolled in their nursing program using a scale from 0 to 100 (0 = absence of stress and 100 = extremely stressed). The average stress rating for both genders was 73 (female 76; male 70). One of the most interesting aspects of the study was asking students to rate their level of stress (using the same rating scale of 0 to 100) after participating in healthy coping activities.

Amazingly, stress levels dropped dramatically; the average level of stress for both genders was 48 (female 50; male 46). This is very important information—it says to me that engaging in coping activities makes a big difference in helping students (and all of us) manage stress.

Stress in Nursing Education

As I think about the impact of stress on productivity and one's psychological well-being, I am reminded of the story a nurse educator recently shared with me. She wore a dejected and sad expression—her shoulders sagged, and she had tears in her eyes. She told me she had recently met with her department chair to discuss her desire to pursue a leadership position within the school of nursing. She had been working hard toward this goal by attending leadership workshops, working with a mentor, reading the works of great leadership scholars, and sharpening her leadership skills on teams and committees. She thought she was poised and ready to take on the challenge of a formal leadership position. When she discussed her intention with her supervisor, the supervisor guffawed—then asked if she was "really serious." She tried to explain how she had made progress on becoming more proficient in her leadership skills, but her supervisor merely shook her head, snickered, and said, "Not a chance."

For some, the painful impact from the stress of incivility remains for years and, in some cases, results in diagnosable mental illnesses. An attendee at one of my civility workshops illustrates this assertion. The attendee—I'll call him Tom—chronicled his prolonged encounters with workplace incivility and asked that his experience (which you can read about in the nearby sidebar) be shared so that others can benefit from his story.

TOM'S STORY

My unhappy journey with workplace incivility began in 2003, when I became the target of a psychologically abusive coworker. I was bullied, ostracized, and made the victim of false and malicious rumors. The pattern of incivility became so extreme

continues

that I reported the problem to my supervisor. I asked for a meeting with my supervisor and the bully. My hope was to discuss the problem and, in a professionally mediated way, find a mutually beneficial and nonpunitive solution. My supervisor agreed to facilitate the meeting, but sadly, the meeting never took place, because the bully refused to attend, and my supervisor did not pursue the issue. About 6 months later, as the situation grew more desperate, I decided to see a mental health professional. I was eventually diagnosed with post-traumatic stress disorder (PTSD), a potentially disabling condition—my diagnosis was directly related to the abusive behavior. After the diagnosis was made, I asked for another facilitated meeting with the bully, and once again, my request remained unaddressed and unresolved. By then, I was dealing with increasing symptoms of PTSD, including high levels of anxiety, eating and sleeping disruptions, nightmares, and hypervigilance. I also experienced a growing sense of dread and isolation, feelings of insecurity and vulnerability, and impaired concentration. Clearly, my condition was beginning to affect my work. I knew I had to find another position. I looked for and found another job. This time I was careful to learn as much as I could about the culture of the organization and the health of the workforce. Today, I am working in a healthy and thriving practice setting. I am still in therapy and still taking medications for my condition—but each day in my new environment, I feel better and better. You see, people living with PTSD do not simply recall what happened to them, they relive it over and over again. My supervisor's inability or refusal to respond to the problem in a responsible and humane manner contributed to my condition. All I wanted was a fair conflict-resolution process with open communication that benefited everyone involved. I believe that dealing with workplace incivility is important—the bully must be held accountable, and if he or she refuses to cooperate, he or she should be reprimanded. To me, incivility is like hand washing—it deserves and needs to be taught, reinforced, and given constant attention and reminders.

Nurse educators are clearly under substantial pressure. Several studies (Clark, 2008a, 2008b, 2013; Clark, Olender, Kenski, & Cardoni, 2013; Clark & Springer, 2010) reveal numerous stressors affecting nursing faculty. Not only do they need to be competent in the scholarly triumvirate of teaching, scholarship, and service, but many nursing faculty are also required to maintain clinical competence. This requirement becomes even more stressful for nursing faculty who are also nurse practitioners (NPs). In addition to their faculty role, our NP colleagues must maintain an active clinical practice and meet certification and renewal requirements to maintain their NP status.

Other stressors include increasingly heavy workloads, workload inequity, issues related to promotion and tenure, and pressure to pursue a doctoral degree. More and more, nursing faculty are being urged (and in some cases required) to complete an advanced degree to maintain their faculty positions. This requisite places tremendous stress on an already strained professorate and creates an almost crippling level of tension as faculty members attempt (like the students they teach and mentor) to juggle the competing demands of school, work, and family. In the original edition of this book, I introduced you to my talented friend and colleague, Max (name used with his express permission), who epitomized many of, if not all, these conditions—Max is a devoted father, who at the time was knee-deep in his doctoral program, a gifted NP, applying for promotion and tenure, juggling a challenging teaching and clinical load, working on a substantial grant application to continue his clinical research, and serving on numerous teams and committees in the school of nursing and beyond. Over the years, I have been constantly amazed at Max's ability to manage his school, work, and family life with such poise and humor. I come back to Max a little later in this chapter.

Faculty members across the nation are also dealing with the challenges of hiring, retaining, and mentoring part-time and adjunct faculty; working with questionable leaders and problematic students; facing low salaries and financial pressures; and keeping pace with up-to-the-minute and ever-changing technology.

Further, when people are stressed, rushed, and unhappy, incivility is a possible outcome (Forni, 2008). For example, most of us would consider ourselves to be civil. However, when we are hurried and feeling overwhelmed or overworked, we are more likely to behave in ways we might not otherwise act. I know that when my stress level is high, and when deadlines are looming, I am more likely to say or do something out of character. Thus, we each need to have a trusted colleague with whom we can talk honestly and who can serve as a barometer when stressful situations arise. If you decide to meet with a friend or colleague, it is best to select a place away from the hectic nature and rapid pace of the work environment. Consider meeting in a neutral, quiet place without interruptions and distractions. Or talk while you walk; our home is located in the high desert of Idaho, surrounded by glorious blankets of wild flowers in the springtime and lovely bird songs from meadowlarks and other happy creatures. What a lovely place to have a conversation with a trusted colleague. Other places might work well, too—a coffee shop, an out-of-the-way classroom, or a conference room where you will be undisturbed.

In addition, often anxiety-producing stressors arise within our nursing programs due to the constant change of curriculum revisions, program additions, course development, committee work, and countless other initiatives that demand our time. These stressors along with personal pressures can provoke uncivil events and encounters. If left unchecked and unaddressed, these disruptive and uncivil behaviors can become a normal pattern and lead to a culture of incivility. The effects of incivility, especially if ingrained, can result in an erosion of self-esteem, damaged relationships, ineffective teamwork, low morale, organizational mistrust, and potential for violence. Moreover, high levels of stress accompanied by poor coping skills can create a potential for conflict and engagement in the "dance of incivility."

The Dance of Incivility—Fostering Civility

In 2008, I introduced a conceptual model to illustrate the intricate and complex "dance" of incivility and civility in nursing education (Clark, 2008a; see Figure 3.1). The conceptual model was later revised to include nursing practice (Clark, Olender, Cardoni, & Kenski, 2011; see Figure 3.2).

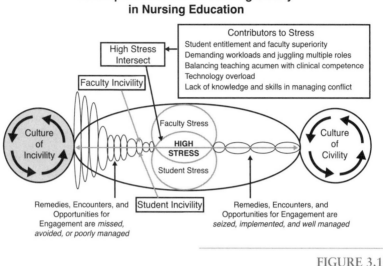

**Conceptual Model for Fostering Civility
in Nursing Education**

FIGURE 3.1

*Conceptual model
for fostering civility in
nursing education.*

The large, oval circle in the center of the model depicts the reciprocal nature of faculty and student encounters. The nucleus of the model indicates a point where high levels of faculty and student stress intersect. This high-stress intersect point is influenced by several factors, including attitudes of student entitlement and faculty superiority, demanding workloads, the juggling of multiple tasks and competing demands, technology and information overload, and lack of the knowledge and skills to effectively manage conflict. Encounters between faculty and students occur constantly and consistently, even when stress levels are low. However, when stress levels are heightened, the encounters can be more intense and can result in threatening behaviors. These behaviors, when combined with heightened stress levels, can increase the potential for incivility (displayed on the left side of the model). The double-sided arrow in the center of the model represents the dynamic continuum of ongoing opportunities for faculty and student engagement to prevent or de-escalate a potentially volatile situation.

The left side of the model illustrates an escalating spiral of incivility that might occur when remedies, encounters, and opportunities to resolve the conflict are missed, avoided, or poorly managed. When these omissions or avoidances occur, the result might be a culture of incivility. Conversely, the right side of the model illustrates how seizing, implementing, and managing well the opportunities for engagement can lead to a culture of civility. When faculty and students work together to resolve conflict, the potential for civility is enhanced, and a safer, more civil learning environment is created. Incivility, whether initiated by faculty, students, or a combination of both, presents opportunities for engagement. When faculty and students effectively communicate and intentionally engage with one another, a culture of civility is achievable.

Conceptual Model for Fostering Civility in Nursing Education (Adapted for Nursing Practice)

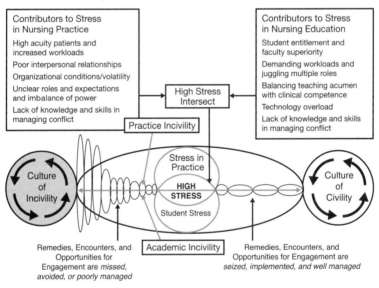

Adapted Clark and Olender © 2010

Clark, C. M., Olender, L., Cardoni, C., & Kenski, D. (2011). Fostering civility in nursing education and practice: Nurse leader perspectives. *Journal of Nursing Administration, 41*(7/8), 324–330.

FIGURE 3.2

Conceptual model for fostering civility in nursing education (adapted for nursing practice).

The conceptual model (adapted for practice) was developed by Clark et al. (2011) to reflect the stressors that contribute to incivility in both nursing education and practice environments. Factors that contribute to stress in nursing practice are similar to the stressors experienced in nursing education, including work overload, unclear roles and expectations, organizational conditions, and a lack of knowledge and skills. Moreover, in both the practice and academic arenas, stress is mitigated by leaders who role-model professionalism and utilize effective communication skills. The importance of modeling effective communication and related education to address incivility cannot be overestimated; it can reduce incivility's incidence and effects, and can assist in fostering cultures of civility.

With this in mind, coping effectively with stress is an important element in preventing incivility. We need to make stress-reduction strategies and self-care measures a part of our daily lives. The American Holistic Nurses Association (2016) recommends several stress-management techniques, including diaphragmatic breathing, progressive muscle relaxation, guided imagery, and mindful meditation. Other stress-reduction techniques include finding quiet time for reflection and contemplation, journaling, yoga, and talking with a trusted person when worries build. Remember my former colleague Max whom I introduced you to earlier in this chapter? I'm delighted to report that Max has successfully defended his doctoral dissertation, received tenure, been promoted to the rank of associate professor, and while he has dealt with an astonishing level of stress, he has achieved amazing results. Max is the master of healthy coping. He manages his stress in numerous healthy ways, including bike rides, river trips, swimming, and just plain hanging out with his son—he is his anchor and an unparalleled source of joy and delight!

Nurse educators also need to role-model and talk about the importance of stress reduction with students. In my role as a nursing professor, each semester, my students and I would engage in an exercise to identify stress-reduction measures we vowed to use throughout the course of the semester. The results of that exercise from one of my Nursing Leadership classes are in the accompanying sidebar.

**STRESS REDUCTION AND SELF-CARE EXERCISE
(DR. CLARK'S NURSING LEADERSHIP CLASS)**

Enjoy family, friends, pets, and supportive people.

Exercise regularly.

Get fresh air and sunshine.

Engage in hobbies and other activities.

Eat healthy, drink lots of water, and get adequate sleep.

Visualize the positive and practice relaxation.

Find quiet time for reflection and contemplation.

Avoid sleeping pills, drugs, and too much alcohol.

When worries start to build up, talk to someone.

Declutter and get organized.

Enjoy your favorite music.

We revisited these exercises throughout the semester and checked in with one another to evaluate our "stress-reducing" aptitude. It helps to have a team of cheerleaders and to know that someone has your back. It is this *esprit de corps* that helps strengthen and reinforce the bonds between and among students and faculty—two groups who will soon become colleagues in a profession with unlimited demands and expectations.

Finishing Touches

Incivility in nursing education and within the greater society is here to stay unless each of us makes a determined and deliberate effort to eradicate it from our midst. It is incumbent upon each of us to raise awareness about the stress associated with incivility and to support one another in our quest to abolish these behaviors and to create a more just and civil society. Doing so will be a challenge, but one we must be prepared to undertake both individually and collectively. If we do not, our spirits and our profession will suffer—an unacceptable and untenable condition.

CIVILITY TIP

Make it a priority to spend time with those you love and with those who love you back. When you interact with family and friends (human and otherwise), you are more likely to lead a balanced, happy life with fewer stress-related symptoms. You are also better at managing your stress when you have a solid social-support system. Even though stress will always be a part of your life and stress management is a work in progress, with practice, you can improve your stress-management capacity and increase your ability to cope with the myriad of life's challenges.

Chapter 4
The "Dance of Incivility and Civility" in Nursing Education

Incivility is like a dance—one dancer leads and the other follows—and sometimes the dancers do both. The steps ebb and flow, and often, the dancers are swept away—moving and gyrating to a frenzied, raucous rhythm, while a sense of defiance seems to take over—and from there, anything can happen. –Cynthia Clark

This chapter discusses:

- Exploring student-to-faculty incivility and faculty-to-student incivility
- Exploring the gap between nursing education and practice
- Exploring faculty-to-faculty incivility
- Exploring student-to-student incivility
- Exploring incivility in the online learning environment

The Dance of Incivility Among Faculty and Students

For more than a decade, I have been deeply intrigued with the study of academic incivility. I am steadfast in my belief that when we understand the issues more completely, we can ultimately develop and implement evidence-based strategies to prevent, address, and minimize incivility. When I first started reading on the topic of incivility, I quickly realized that conflict in higher education has almost always existed; however, when I read Boice's (1996) seminal work on student incivility published 20 years ago, I was not only intrigued with his findings but moreover believed that this topic was one requiring extensive and ongoing examination. My quest to learn as much as possible about academic incivility in general, and in nursing education in particular, eventually led me to the work of Feldman (2001), who presented an eloquent taxonomy of uncivil student behaviors that ranged from annoyances to terrorism, intimidation, and threats. He described such annoyances as sleeping in class, not paying attention, leaving class early, and misusing cellphones. Classroom terrorists demonstrated more disruptive behaviors, such as dominating class and showing a clear disdain or intolerance for others' points of view. Intimidating behaviors included making threats to others, intentionally tarnishing reputations, and bad-mouthing faculty through anonymous teaching evaluations. Threats of violence made up the final category of the taxonomy and included the most destructive forms of incivility, such as students physically attacking other students or faculty. Fortunately, violence is rare in higher education, but none of us will ever forget the lives lost in such terrible tragedies as the shooting deaths at the University of Arizona in 2002, Virginia Tech in 2007, Northern Illinois University in 2008, Oikos University in 2012, and Northern Arizona University and Umpqua Community College in 2015—just to mention a very few.

The University of Arizona shooting was pivotal in shaping the trajectory of my life—both personally and professionally. The shooter in this tragedy committed a premeditated act of violence, terrorizing the campus, the community, and the nation. Prior to the shooting, the gunman authored a 26-page manifesto detailing his rage at the University of Arizona nursing faculty and mailed it to the *Arizona Daily Star* shortly before his death. He tried to justify his actions by claiming that he had been unfairly treated by faculty in his attempts to succeed in his nursing program. This manifesto prompted widespread discussion and debate on violence in higher education in general, and nursing education in particular. I was determined to learn more about preventing these tragic events from ever happening again. How naïve I was—as campus shootings continued.

The shootings at Northern Illinois University occurred in my native state—and at the university my niece was attending at the time. One of my faculty colleagues at Boise State University was also from Illinois, and I remember distinctly to this day how she raced from her office to mine exclaiming, "Cindy, shots fired at NIU, shots fired at NIU!" I remember being gripped with anxiety and fear, then quickly jumped online to follow the horrific scene as it unfolded.

The shootings at Umpqua Community College happened just a stone's throw away from my sister's home in Oregon, where several members of her church group were attending classes—and just a few hours' drive from our home in Boise. Later, in June 2016, a brilliant engineering professor was brutally gunned down on the campus of UCLA. The shooter was armed with two semi-automatic handguns and carrying extra magazines. Sadly, this storyline has become so common and cliché that this terrible event went largely unnoticed and was tragically short-lived on the news cycle.

Surely, none will ever forget the massacre that occurred on December 14, 2012, at Sandy Hook Elementary School in Newtown, Connecticut, when a gunman fatally shot 20 schoolchildren and 6 adult staff members. The incident was the deadliest mass shooting at a high school or grade school in U.S. history. Since the Newtown tragedy, *Everytown for Gun Safety*, an advocacy group, has been tracking school shootings in the United States. At this writing, there have been 186 shootings on school campuses—84 of them occurring at colleges and universities. This is a staggering and sobering number (2016).

Fortunately, the majority of uncivil student behaviors are considered low-intensity or mildly disruptive behaviors, such as talking in class, arriving late or leaving class early, or texting or misusing computers and other media devices. However, more disruptive behaviors of student incivility are also being reported—such behaviors as showing disdain toward faculty while they are teaching, faculty being challenged and confronted during class, and students making rude or disparaging remarks. More extreme behaviors, such as students making threats of violence and making statements about having access to weapons, are far less common, but unfortunately, these behaviors are increasing.

More than a decade ago, much of what I was reading focused more on student incivility and less on uncivil faculty behaviors. Then I came to appreciate the excellent contributions to the literature published by Morrissette (2001), who stressed the importance of faculty using respectful communication in dealing with students, engaging them in meaningful learning experiences, and role-modeling professional behavior. Similarly, Carbone (1999) had suggested that faculty increase their accessibility and availability to students and be more transparent with students about the expectations of desired classroom behavior as well as the subsequent consequences for incivility. About the same time, Braxton and Bayer (1999, 2004) identified seven empirically based uncivil faculty behaviors that undermined student learning and the teaching-learning environment. Some of the behaviors included condescending negativism (defined as treating students in a condescending and demeaning way), being unprepared for class, failing to give equal consideration to all students, using inconsistent grading, and showing preferential treatment toward certain students. The authors concluded that when faculty members violate these norms, it negatively affects the teaching-learning environment and can provoke retaliation of uncivil behavior by students toward others.

I also read everything I could about academic incivility in nursing education. Beginning in the early 2000s, Lashley and De Meneses (2001) researched the extent to which certain problematic student behaviors existed in nursing education, how the behaviors were addressed, and how specific student behaviors compared to 5 years earlier. The authors surveyed 611 nursing programs in the United States and found that the level of uncivil student behaviors ranged from mild to serious. Less disruptive behaviors included tardiness and leaving class early and progressed to more serious behaviors, such as yelling at faculty in the classroom and clinical settings and making objectionable physical contact. The authors also reported that the level of student incivility had increased over a 5-year period and called for a national forum to address the problem.

Shortly after, Luparell (2003) conducted a qualitative study to examine faculty members' perception of student incivility in nursing education. Twenty-one nursing faculty participated in the study, and all had experienced at least one uncivil encounter with a student. For some faculty, the incidents of student incivility were aggressive and severe, resulting in psychological distress and feelings of self-doubt about their teaching abilities. Two faculty members incurred significant financial costs associated with reconciling the uncivil event, and three others cited student incivility as one of the reasons for their departure and retirement from teaching.

In many cases, faculty did not report the uncivil student behavior to college administrators for fear of losing their jobs, because student input on faculty evaluations is closely tied to progress toward promotion and tenure. Faculty were also concerned about a sense of threat to self, loved ones, and personal belongings. In instances when faculty made administrators aware of the uncivil encounters, many reported a disturbing lack of support. When faculty members were supported, many perceived the grievance procedure as heavily weighted in favor of students and described feeling like they were on trial (Luparell, 2003).

After reading Luparell's doctoral dissertation on faculty encounters with student incivility, I decided to contact her directly. Imagine my delight and surprise when her email response popped up on my computer screen. We engaged in a thought-provoking discussion about the state of incivility in nursing education. I was very interested in her findings, yet I was also curious about a question that had been bothering me: If faculty are reporting uncivil encounters with students, what might students have to say about uncivil encounters with faculty?

So I kept reading and wondering. In 2003, Thomas asked nursing students about their experiences with faculty incivility. Students were frustrated with unexpected changes in clinical schedules, inconsistencies in the course syllabus, and nursing faculty who "seem to make up the rules as they go." These encounters often resulted in student anger, which in turn led to disrupted student-faculty relationships, problematic learning environments, and increased stress levels among students and faculty. Hall (2004) had also begun to identify the negative impact of uncivil faculty behaviors on students and suggested that nursing faculty might contribute to dehumanizing conditions that could result in student distress and desperation.

After delving into these important studies, I realized I was on to something and began to study academic incivility in earnest. I realized that we needed a quantitative instrument to measure the type and frequency of incivility with large sample sizes in nursing education and from both student and faculty perspectives. So, in 2004, I designed the Incivility in Nursing Education (INE) survey to measure this phenomenon.

I conducted one of my first studies in 2005 using the INE survey (Clark, Farnsworth, & Landrum, 2009). The INE survey is based on two different instruments designed to measure faculty and student incivility in higher education: the "Defining Classroom Incivility" survey designed by the Center for Survey Research at Indiana University (2000) and the "Student Classroom Incivility Measure" (known as the SCIM-Part C), where students were asked to rate uncivil faculty behaviors in the classroom (Hanson, 2000). For a detailed description about the development and psychometric properties of the INE, please refer to Clark, Farnsworth, and Landrum (2009).

I conducted the study in one school of nursing in the northwestern part of the United States, and it consisted of two parts: a quantitative portion and a qualitative portion, where we examined faculty and student perceptions of and experience with incivility in nursing education, contributing factors, and effective ways to address incivility (Clark & Springer, 2007a, 2007b). Both groups perceived incivility as a moderate (60.2%) to serious (8.7%) problem in the nursing academic environment, and the majority of respondents (61.9%) believed that students were more likely to engage in uncivil behaviors than faculty. We found that the most frequently occurring uncivil student behaviors were students arriving late to class, holding distracting conversations, leaving early, being unprepared, and acting bored or apathetic. We also reported on threatening behaviors demonstrated by students, which included challenges to faculty credibility, general taunts or disrespect to faculty and other students, inappropriate emails to other students, and vulgarity directed at faculty. These are concerning results, because threatening behaviors have the potential to lead to aggression and violence.

The qualitative findings were also illuminating. We asked faculty and students to describe how and why students contribute to incivility in nursing education. The responses were grouped into two major categories:

in-class disruptions and out-of-class disruptions. The in-class student disruptions included students openly challenging faculty, dominating class discussion, making rude gestures, and misusing computers and other media devices by talking and text messaging. Out-of-class disruptions included students "bad-mouthing" other students or faculty and sending negative or inappropriate emails regarding classmates and faculty. We also asked students to consider the potential causes for incivility in nursing education, and we discovered that, once again, stress was a major contributor. Other perceived causes included use of distance learning and the virtual classroom, where students can be somewhat anonymous; lack of faculty credibility and responsiveness; faculty arrogance; and a lack of immediacy to address incivility. Subsequent studies (Altmiller, 2012; Clark, 2008a, 2008b; Clark et al., 2012) also reveal that stress plays a role in the display of uncivil behaviors in the academic environment.

In the same two-part study (Clark & Springer, 2007a, 2007b), we found faculty were also reported to be uncivil to students and sometimes to one another. Uncivil faculty behaviors included faculty belittling or taunting students; using sarcasm, humiliation, intimidation, or profanity; being distant, inflexible, or rigid toward others; and punishing the class for one student's misbehavior. We also reported perceived threatening behaviors committed by faculty. These behaviors included challenging other faculty's knowledge or credibility, general taunts or disrespect toward students or other faculty, sending inappropriate emails to students, and making harassing comments directed at students.

In the qualitative portion of the study, several themes emerged regarding uncivil faculty behaviors, including faculty being condescending, using poor teaching skills or methods, engaging in poor communication, acting superior or arrogant, criticizing students, and threatening to fail students.

Perhaps most importantly, the student and faculty respondents were asked to suggest strategies to address incivility and to improve the culture of the teaching-learning environment. Ideas they offered included pursuing a swift, immediate response to incivility; establishing codes and standards of behavior; implementing policies to address the uncivil behavior; and conducting open and ongoing forums to resolve conflicts among faculty and students.

This study was immediately followed by an in-depth qualitative analysis of student perceptions of faculty incivility. I was intensely curious about stories that students might relate regarding their experiences with faculty incivility. I wondered whether students shared some of the same perceptions and suffered from some of the same psychological and physiological influences the faculty experienced after uncivil student encounters.

The next year, I published a phenomenological study describing nursing students' lived experiences with faculty incivility (Clark, 2006). I conducted in-person interviews with the students and in one case spent a considerable amount of time perusing a journal kept by one of the students throughout the course of his nursing education experience. The journal provided an in-depth chronological account of one student's experience with faculty incivility over time. After interviewing each student, I analyzed more than 250 typed pages of transcription to organize student narratives into themes and to create a succinct summary of the students' individual and collective experience with faculty incivility.

One of the best parts of the study was meeting and getting to know the participants. Each student had a story to tell, and all were eager to share them with me. I would like to introduce you to two of the students who participated in the study. One of the participants—I'll call her Danielle for this discussion—was a 34-year-old nurse who progressed through three nursing programs in pursuit of her bachelor of science in nursing (BSN) degree. Danielle began her nursing education in a licensed practical nurse (LPN) program and quickly earned her associate degree and eventually her bachelor's degree in the span of 7 years. Danielle was thrilled when she was accepted to the nursing program, but her enthusiasm vanished starting on her first day of clinical:

I loved going to class. I loved everybody. I just soaked it all in. I thought the whole thing was absolutely wonderful and I was going to be the happiest nurse in the world. But, I had some self-esteem issues. I took criticism personally. I was 27, but I felt like I was 18. It [the uncivil act] happened my very first day on the medical surgical floor. I was given a patient who was diabetic, and we hadn't studied diabetes in class. The instructor asked me about the patient's blood sugar levels and insulin dosages. I didn't know what blood sugars were, and I didn't know what insulin was. But I remember writing the blood sugars in my notes because I knew it was probably important. She [the instructor] was so gruff and rough that I totally went blank. She just kept getting tougher and tougher with me, and she wouldn't explain anything to me. She told me I would never be a good nurse and she walked away. More than anything in the whole world, I wanted to be a good nurse, and when she said that, it just broke my heart. I had several incidents with that same instructor in that clinical rotation. After that incident happened, I went home bawling. I wasn't going to let anybody see me crying, and I definitely wasn't going to let the instructor see me crying. They would think I was too weak and would try to weed me out. I cried all the way home.

Danielle described many episodes of incivility, but with incredible perseverance, she graduated and eventually completed her degree.

Another student participant, whom I will call David for this example, was a 49-year-old nurse in the final semester of his master's in nursing program. Nursing was a second career for David, and he had been practicing nursing for the past 10 years. He was a salesman, worked as a mechanic, and worked several odd jobs in the early part of his adult life. He loved nursing and enjoyed making a difference in his patients' lives. He considered himself a caring and skilled nurse.

David expressed his displeasure with perceived gender bias as he described how his papers were graded differently than those of his female classmates:

The problem was her grading style. She would take something small like a comma to task where other papers were just blatantly very poorly written or redundant or inconsistent and there wasn't a mark on them. And here I had a simple comma out of place. She would write in big black ink with a couple of exclamation points behind it. And I'm like what in the heck is that all about? She would actually write on the female students' papers, "I'm not taking off points for punctuation," where mine would say, "Bam, here's 10 points off for a comma." You could look at the papers and see that it was just ridiculous.

Without exception, each student described the emotional impact he or she experienced as a result of an uncivil faculty encounter. Interestingly, the amount of time that elapsed from the uncivil faculty encounter to the telling of one's story did nothing to diminish the damaging impact of the event. At the time of the interviews, participants reported that they still felt traumatized by their experiences. Two of them contacted me after their interviews to say that they felt better after telling their stories.

I derived several major themes related to faculty incivility from the student stories—including faculty making demeaning and belittling remarks, treating students unfairly or subjectively, and pressuring students to conform. When I asked students how the uncivil encounters affected them, three major themes emerged: the students felt traumatized, they felt powerless and helpless, and they felt angry. Many students related stories of being humiliated (often publicly) by faculty. Danielle wrote:

> *The professor scolded me because I used two assessment sheets. She told me I wasted paper by using two sheets. She really ripped me apart. She really let me have it, and she did it in front of other students. The other students who were there, just stood there. I took her scolding and said, "This will never happen again," but inside I was ready to burst. I felt like I couldn't do anything right. I hated clinical after that.*

Following the completion of my study, I crafted a succinct summary of the students' experiences with faculty incivility; it appears in the accompanying sidebar.

STUDY SUMMARY (CLARK, 2006)

Students subjected to faculty incivility described vivid accounts of their experiences with faculty incivility in nursing education. Some students were still reeling from their uncivil encounters with faculty, even when the event occurred several months to several years prior to the interview. Uncivil faculty behaviors reported by students included faculty demeaning and belittling students, treating them unfairly, and pressuring students to conform to unreasonable faculty demands. Other faculty behaviors included gender bias, violation of due process, subjective grading, "weeding students out," and threatening to fail them if they didn't conform to rigid faculty demands. Students reported that it is often "the little things" (persistent over time) that faculty members do to provoke student anger and frustration.

For some, the impact of the uncivil faculty encounters was so emotional that students experienced psychological and physiological symptoms. Students reported feeling traumatized, helpless, powerless, and angry. Some reported losing sleep, pacing at night, arguing with family and friends, and feeling legitimate guilt about cheating to pass nursing courses. The students felt inferior to faculty and caught in a "no-win" power struggle with little possibility for successful resolution. They described a sense of powerlessness and being at a disadvantage primarily because of the power differential between faculty and students and the faculty member's abuse of authority and rank. Students felt they "had too much to lose" by confronting faculty on their uncivil behavior. If they pursued the matter with faculty or other educational administrators, they worried they would be failed in a course or, even worse, be expelled from the nursing program. In some cases, the students did address the incivility with faculty only to be treated with even greater indignity and disrespect. In most cases, students accepted the uncivil treatment as part of the "hoop jumping" required to complete the program. Students described "playing the game" and keeping their head down to complete the program and to get on with their lives, because they had a significant amount of money and time invested in their education.

The students who "made it" were supported by family and friends, but supportive and nurturing nursing faculty made a larger and more lasting impact on the students' decision to stay or leave the program. The struggle to make sense of the incivility leaves the students feeling ambivalent at best. Some reported wishing they had confronted the faculty about the incivility but weighed that decision against the consequences of doing so, which they perceived to be quite grave. In all but one case, the students felt more capable of dealing with future acts of incivility

continues

in other arenas of their lives subsequent to their experiences with uncivil faculty behaviors in their nursing education. In one case, a student felt that the level of faculty incivility was so extreme and pervasive that the experience caused some of his classmates to compromise their integrity and ethics and go into a "survival mode" to make it through the program. This student believed that his classmates were willing to sacrifice their personal integrity for their own perceived well-being.

Soon after conducting the previous studies, I used the INE survey with a large national sample of nursing students and faculty to gather their perceptions about the types and frequency of incivility in nursing education, major contributors to incivility, and, most importantly, evidence-based strategies to address the problem. The respondents included 306 nursing students and 194 nursing faculty from 41 states, who reported incivility to be a moderate to severe problem in nursing education. The most frequently experienced uncivil student behaviors included students arriving late for class, holding distracting conversations, leaving early, being unprepared, and creating tensions by dominating class discussion. The qualitative findings included students misusing cellphones and computers; engaging in side conversations and dominating class; making rude remarks; and using sarcasm, vulgarity, and cyberbullying tactics. Other major themes included students pressuring faculty until they acquiesced to student demands and "bad mouthing" other students, faculty, and the nursing program. The two main contributing factors were stress and a sense of student entitlement. Students complained of stress associated with demanding workloads, academic competition, and the feeling that they were compelled to cheat to compete for grades, scholarships, and placement in the program.

Faculty reported feeling stressed due to burnout from demanding workloads, high faculty turnover, competing demands, and exposure to incivility. I found faculty superiority, arrogance, and an abuse of authority over students to be potentially destructive behaviors. When faculty exert their position and power over students, assume a "know-it-all" attitude, and arbitrarily threaten to fail or dismiss students, the possibility for incivility increases.

When you look at these attitudes of student entitlement and faculty superiority a bit closer, it becomes clear that heightened stress levels among faculty and students, accompanied by negative attitudes of faculty superiority and student entitlement, increase the potential for incivility in nursing education.

When an attitude of student entitlement is present, you might find it represented in the following ways: Students might assume a "know-it-all" attitude and a consumer mentality, believing that they are owed an education and believing that because they paid for an "A," they should receive an "A." This sense of entitlement is also reflected in some students' refusal to accept personal responsibility. Some blame others, deflect accountability, and make excuses for their shortcomings or lack of academic achievement. One nursing faculty put it this way: "I had a student come up to me in clinical and demand that I give her an 'A' because she paid for it, and therefore deserved it. Besides, she needed to maintain a high GPA to keep her financial aid." This sense of entitlement and arrogance, though infrequent, can be very disruptive to faculty-student relationships and the overall teaching-learning environment. However, we need to remember in some cases, what might appear to be a sense of student entitlement might, in fact, be the students' attempt to become a conscientious consumer of education in a competitive market. A student might have a legitimate concern about a faculty member's decision and behave in what looks like an "entitled" manner, and this concern might be mistaken for entitlement (Achacoso, 2006). Faculty need to consider the context of the situation and determine the intent of the behavior to enhance the likelihood of successful resolution of the conflict or disagreement (Clark, 2008a).

In many of my studies, I have also found that when faculty members are stressed, they are more likely to exhibit uncivil behaviors and, moreover, demonstrate an attitude of superiority by exerting their position or power over students, setting unrealistic expectations, threatening to fail or dismiss students, or devaluing students' previous life work and academic experience. This sense of superiority can have a negative impact not only on relationships but also on the learning environment and the entire campus community. A sense of faculty superiority can have devastating effects—and when such superiority is paired with a student sense of entitlement, there will be no winners. Ultimately, high levels of stress and poor coping, coupled with attitudes of student entitlement and faculty superiority, can create a potential for conflict and engagement in the dance of incivility.

One of the most chilling findings in my civility work involves students' disclosure of academic dishonesty and cheating. Most of the stories have less to do with cheating in the classroom than they do with cheating in the clinical area. Fortunately, this type of cheating in the practice setting is not common; however, the effects can be far-reaching and seriously impact patient quality of care and patient safety. For example, students have admitted falsifying information in patients' medical records. In one case, a student described how he did not have time to take a patient's blood pressure or measure a blood sugar level, so he made up the information and recorded it in the medical record. Another student divulged that she claimed to have changed a sterile dressing on a patient when in fact she had not. These revelations are troubling and inexcusable. Students rationalized their behavior by explaining that if they admitted their indiscretions, they might be failed or dismissed from the program and that the fierce competition for nursing-program placement justified their abhorrent behavior.

Overall, the Clark studies (2008a, 2008b) concluded that incivility in nursing education often results in psychological and physiological distress in both faculty and students and can negatively impact the academic environment. Strategies for addressing incivility included engaging in direct communication and working together to create a culture of civility by establishing, disseminating, and enforcing policies to address incivility, co-creating classroom norms, providing syllabi reviews and focused orientation programs, and providing ongoing education and public forums to discuss effective solutions for preventing and dealing with the problem.

Del Prato (2013) found similar results when exploring students' lived experiences with faculty incivility in associate degree nursing education. She found that faculty incivility comprised four interrelated experiences: verbally abusive and demeaning experiences, favoritism and subjective evaluation, rigid expectations for perfection and time management, and targeting and weeding-out practices. These experiences resulted in student disillusionment with both faculty and the nursing profession. Altmiller

(2012) found that students' perceptions of faculty incivility included demonstrating unprofessional behavior, using poor communication techniques, and exerting power over students. The author suggested that clearly communicating course-related information, promptly addressing problematic behaviors, maintaining classroom decorum, and setting a positive example of civility can help improve faculty-student relationships and the teaching-learning environment.

Mott (2014) conducted a qualitative, phenomenological study describing students lived experiences with faculty bullying behaviors. The findings were consistent with other studies on faculty incivility toward students. In the Mott study, faculty incivility caused students to feel an array of emotions including anger, fear, sadness, frustration, and a sense of diminished self-confidence. Faculty incivility also had a negative impact on the students' ability to learn. Participants also reported that faculty incivility/disrespect prompted a desire to respond in kind in disrespectful ways. This finding is consistent with a study conducted in the People's Republic of China (Clark et al., 2012) where students described the reciprocal nature of incivility as a "careless collision" between faculty and students.

Intervention studies are needed to prevent and address incivility and to foster healthy academic and practice environments. I referred to the following study (Clark, 2011) in Chapter 2. It was an amazing experience to be contacted by the director of a nursing school whose program had been cited by the state board of nursing (BON) for numerous "incivility" infractions, including student, faculty, and practice-based incivility indiscretions. The BON required the nursing program to develop and implement a clearly defined set of expectations, strategies, and written policies "to enhance student-faculty relationships and to improve the culture of academic civility" (Clark, 2011, p. 98). Many complaints centered on the type, level, and frequency of incivility occurring in the nursing program and extending throughout the practice environments. The BON required that significant improvements be demonstrated within 6 months of the report; otherwise, the program would be closed. I led a broad-based initiative to address the problem. We used an ambitious intervention plan with an action research approach to conduct pre- and post-intervention assessments, a series of workshops with faculty and students, and individual and group-based strategies.

First, I had the faculty and students complete a pre-intervention assessment using the INE survey (Clark, Farnsworth, & Landrum, 2009) to measure the perceived type, level, and frequency of uncivil student and faculty behaviors within the nursing program. The majority of the participants (82%) perceived incivility to be a moderate to serious problem. Students identified several uncivil student behaviors, including students holding distracting conversations, acting bored or apathetic, and arriving late to class. Faculty reported uncivil student behaviors, including students arriving late to class, holding distracting conversations, being unprepared for class, and leaving class early. Students reported several uncivil faculty behaviors, including faculty being cold and distant, making condescending remarks, refusing or being reluctant to answer questions, threatening to fail students, making rude gestures or behaviors, and punishing the entire class for one student's misbehavior. Faculty noted similar frequently occurring uncivil faculty behaviors, including faculty exerting superiority, threatening to fail students, not allowing open discussion, being inflexible and rigid, and being unavailable outside class.

After we had a good reading on the type and frequency of uncivil faculty and student behavior, I conducted a series of workshops with both groups. We used Heinrich's four-step approach (2010b, 2011) for negotiating collaborative partnership agreements to create a sense of trust and to develop a set of working norms. We discussed the problem of incivility in depth and developed and implemented several group and individual strategies targeted at fostering civility. After the strategies were implemented, I conducted the post-intervention assessment. We needed to determine whether the types and level of incivility had improved. Remarkably, on nearly every measure, we found improvement. Most notably, the perceived level of moderate to serious incivility dropped from 82% to 74%; and 50% of students reported an improvement in overall civility. Nearly all uncivil student behaviors dropped (improved), and four of the six uncivil faculty behaviors dropped (improved).

On the post-intervention assessment, I asked both groups for their opinions regarding the most effective individual strategies to foster civility. Students reported the most effective individual strategies as being respectful and prepared, communicating needs, and clarifying faculty expectations. Faculty reported greeting students, listening, and providing positive feedback as the most effective individual strategies. The most effective group strategies used by students included following classroom and clinical norms, assisting others, and working toward a common goal of civility and respect. Effective group strategies used by faculty were engaging in a meaningful dialogue about civility, developing vision and mission statements, becoming more active members of the faculty, and treating one another with respect. Despite the ambitious time frame to show improvement in the type, level, and frequency of faculty and student incivility, we managed to achieve modest gains. Since conducting this intervention study, I have worked with several nursing programs to facilitate the transformation of their workplace culture. In nearly every case, I have used empirical measures as pre-/post-assessments to determine the program's specific issues to carefully implement an evidence-based action plan based on the program's unique and individualized needs. Chapter 7 explains this approach in greater detail.

While I was conducting the studies described above, others performed important studies—notably the studies on "connectivity" in the online learning environment (Rieck & Crouch, 2007) and on legal perspectives and strategies to handle academic incivility (Suplee, Lachman, Siebert, & Anselmi, 2008). The former study examined perceptions of "connectiveness" and civility in online nursing courses and provided strategies to promote civility with peers, including face-to-face instruction, meeting at the beginning of the semester, encouraging discussion boards and chats, and improving pedagogical course design and group work. The latter study examined highly prevalent and typical examples of incivility and discussed legal perspectives and strategies to handle incivility. The authors of this study suggested various ways to foster civility, including developing administrative policies, enacting faculty development, and setting ground rules. Both studies broadened the body of research on incivility in nursing education and provided helpful solutions to address the problem.

Soon after, Marchiondo, Marchiondo, and Lasiter (2010) explored the most common locations of faculty incivility and the overall effects of faculty incivility on senior baccalaureate nursing students and the impact on program satisfaction. The researchers developed and utilized the Nursing Education Environment Survey (NEES), which included questions regarding program satisfaction, optimism, and incivility. Results revealed that the majority of respondents (88%) experienced at least one instance of uncivil behavior; while 40% experienced incivility from one faculty member, a nearly equal amount (43%) experienced incivility from two different faculty members. The students reported that the highest frequency of incivility occurred in the classroom (60%), followed next by the clinical setting (50%), and least frequently in the laboratory (10%). The authors of this study noted a relationship between faculty incivility and program satisfaction. The most common actions taken by students experiencing faculty incivility fell into the following categories: talking about it with a friend, partner, or spouse; talking to classmates about it; and putting up with it. Students were least likely to make formal complaints to the university, make excuses so the instructor would leave them alone, or assume that the instructor meant well.

In a subsequent publication, and as part of the initial study, Lasiter, Marchiondo, and Marchiondo (2012) asked students to describe their worst experience of faculty incivility. The students described four major categories: incivility "in front of someone" (in the presence of others), "talked to others about me," "made to feel stupid," and "felt belittled." These uncivil faculty behaviors had a significant effect on students by increasing pressure on academic and clinical performance and decreasing program satisfaction and retention. The authors called for the development of guidelines for preventing and managing faculty-student incivility, encouraging students to take an active role in addressing the problem, and instituting processes to report the problem without fear of retaliation.

Luparell (2011) wrote a compelling article on the effects of incivility on nurses, patients, and healthcare organizations. The author suggests that targeted conversations between academic and clinical settings can help in reaching a solution on ways to address incivility and bullying. Luparell provides some very important points, including whether a more aggressive assessment of individuals entering nursing programs should be undertaken, where the emphasis on student learning and evaluation would best be placed, how well staff nurses are prepared to participate in the educational process, and how students are socialized into the profession.

Bridging the Gap Between Nursing Education and Practice

Incivility not only negatively impacts the academic environment, but the clinical environment as well. Kerber, Woith, Jenkins, and Schafer Astroth (2015) conducted a qualitative study to explore the impact of incivility in the practice environment on new nurses and patients. Participants described uncivil interactions involving new and experienced nurses, nurse leaders, physicians, patients, and families. They also described how uncivil interactions negatively impacted their emotional, professional, and physical well-being—and most disturbing, the harmful effects of incivility on patient care. The authors emphasized the crucial role professional staff development plays in promoting a culture of civility by raising awareness, supporting new nurses as they adjust to professional practice, and helping healthcare workers cope with incivility through the use of simulation to practice civil responses during uncivil encounters.

Babenko-Mould and Laschinger (2014) conducted a quantitative study to examine the relationship between nursing students' exposure to various forms of incivility in their clinical learning environments and their experience of burnout and emotional exhaustion. Using the Cortina Incivility Scale (CIS) and the Emotional Exhaustion (EE) and Cynicism (C) subscales of the Maslach Burnout Inventory-General Survey (MBI-GS), the authors measured nursing student experiences of incivility from clinical instructors, nursing staff, and other healthcare professionals and the relationship to burnout and emotional exhaustion. Results from the study revealed that the detrimental effects of incivility within nursing students' clinical learning environments were associated with burnout and emotional exhaustion, and that the influence of incivility from nurses was particularly strong. The authors stressed the important need for nurse educators to address the problem of incivility during the students' nursing education experience. This is particularly important because uncivil work environments contribute to poor morale, decreased productivity, and greater job turnover.

A few years ago, I conducted a study (Clark, Olender, Cardoni, & Kenski, 2011) in which I asked 174 leaders in nursing practice (CNOs, administrators, supervisors, and managers) their best advice to bridge the gap between nursing education and practice. Specifically, I asked nurse leaders how nursing education and nursing practice can work together to foster civility in healthcare organizations. Their top responses included crafting a collective vision of civility, constructing a shared nursing curriculum, improving communication and partnerships, integrating civility into the nursing curriculum, and establishing codes of conduct and policies for civility.

This study (and others) cemented my desire to explore effective ways for nursing practice and education to work together. In 2015, I had the high honor and privilege to be selected as one of the co-chairs by the American Nurses Association (ANA) to assist in authoring the position statement on workplace incivility, bullying, and violence (ANA, 2015b). In early fall 2014, the ANA issued a nationwide call for nurses to serve on the professional panel; incredibly, more than 500 members expressed interest. It was the largest applicant pool for a professional issues panel ever assembled. The panel included four co-chairs, 24 steering committee members, 441 advisory committee members, and ANA staff members. Our goal was to develop a strong, comprehensive, evidence-based position statement on incivility, bullying, and workplace violence to help nurses and employers across the healthcare continuum (including practice and academia) deal with these problems and to promote and sustain healthy workplaces. While the position statement was written specifically for nurses and employers, the panel took great care to make sure the statement was relevant to other healthcare providers and stakeholders. The statement articulates individual and shared responsibilities to foster healthy work environments and to implement best practices to prevent and address incivility, bullying, and violence to ensure optimal outcomes across the healthcare continuum.

Other authors (Trépanier, Fernet, Austin, & Boudrias, 2016) conducted an integrative review of the antecedents of workplace bullying for registered nurses and subsequently integrated the antecedents into a theoretical model. Based on the integrative review of 12 studies, the authors identified four main categories of work-related antecedents of workplace bullying: job characteristics, quality of interpersonal relationships, leadership styles, and organizational culture.

In the job characteristics category, seven characteristics were found to be significant correlates of bullying in nurses. Workplace bullying was positively related to workload, organizational constraints, and bad and stressful work situations and negatively related to job control, promotional opportunities, reward, and structural empowerment. In other words, manageable workload, job control, and reward were negatively correlated with reports of nurse bullying. Nurses experiencing high levels of bullying reported significantly higher workload and organizational constraints and significantly less job control and promotional opportunities. Further, "in situations of stress, nurses are less tolerant and more prone to lash out at others through negative behaviors" (Trépanier et al., 2016, p. 90).

Regarding the quality of interpersonal relationships, workplace bullying was negatively linked to work group cohesion, social support (from the supervisor and mentor), communication and trust within teams, and a sense of community at work as well as shared values. Bullying was also positively related to the presence of cliques. In addition, a lack of trust and poor communication were also significantly related to the presence of nurse bullying. The authors suggest that poor communication and a lack of cooperation and trust may prevent employees from openly discussing their problems, which may lead to accumulated anger and frustration and ultimately further conflicts. Moreover, individuals in a position of authority (i.e., supervisor or mentor) may be uniquely qualified to provide support and ways to address conflict in a constructive manner (Trépanier et al., 2016).

In the category of leadership styles, the authors found that authentic leadership fosters a climate of trust and positive interpersonal relationships. Authentic leaders also promote constructive ways to manage conflict based on cooperation rather than competition (Trépanier et al., 2016).

In the final category of organizational culture, Trépanier et al. suggested that bullying is more likely to occur when it becomes part of the organizational norms and values, especially if the behavior is allowed to persist, and worse, when it is rewarded and viewed as part of the job. Work environments where decisions are made unfairly and where advantages and rewards are distributed unjustly are more likely to foster bullying behaviors (Trépanier et al., 2016).

Castronovo, Pullizzi, and Evans (2016) also conducted a review of the literature on nurse bullying and proposed a unique solution to address the problem. The authors suggested that a national standardized measurement tool similar to the Hospital Consumer Assessment of Healthcare Providers and Systems (HCAHPS) be developed and implemented to measure nurse's perspectives of workplace bullying. They further propose that results from the survey would be factored into the calculation of the value-based incentive payment program, allowing healthcare institutions to be incentivized to measure, address, and successfully resolve the problem of nurse bullying.

These are compelling and thought-provoking studies that require deeper and ongoing investigation. In fact, it would be interesting to see how findings from these works compare to incivility and bullying in nursing programs. Some studies have been conducted to assess various interventions in nursing education. For example, Jenkins, Kerber, and Woith (2013) conducted an exploratory mixed-methods study to test whether participation in a journal club was an effective intervention to change civility perceptions among nursing students. The authors found that participation in the journal club changed students' attitudes and behaviors regarding civility, including students' refusing to participate in uncivil behavior, being more supportive toward others, and attempting to prevent or avoid incivility.

In a more recent study (Doherty, Landry, Pate, & Reid, 2016), the authors implemented and evaluated the effectiveness of a communication competency educational program to improve students' advocacy behaviors. Portions of the TeamSTEPPS curriculum were used as an experiential learning strategy to improve communication and teamwork within the practice environment. The authors described how the intentional use of competency-based communication models used within the context of Knowles' Adult Learning Theory had a positive impact on the students' ability to advocate for themselves and their patients. Results from pre- to post-intervention indicated the importance of communication competency education when advocating for themselves or for their patients.

While these studies continue, it is my fervent belief that nurse educators play a key role in preparing nursing students to prevent, identify, and address incivility in the workplace. Another promising approach (Clark, Ahten, & Macy, 2012) involves the use of live actors and Problem-Based Learning techniques to simulate uncivil encounters in the workplace where students can role-play, discuss, and practice cognitively rehearsed scripts to effectively address incivility in the practice setting. After using the combination of role-play and cognitive rehearsal, the authors conducted a follow-up study 10 months later, and found that the participants in the previous study reported being better prepared to address incivility as newly graduated nurses (Clark, Ahten, & Macy, 2014).

This study inspired another investigation using a mixed methods approach and a simulated scenario with newly graduated nurses to explore the potential impact of uncivil communication on patient care and tested whether an intervention using cognitive rehearsal could effectively mitigate the negative effects of workplace incivility. This first of its kind study involved actors using a verbatim script to portray an uncivil nurse-to-nurse encounter during a patient hand-off report. At strategic points throughout the simulated experience, we measured the effects of stress on the nurse receiving the hand-off report using biomarkers found in saliva, heart rate, blood pressure readings, and self-assessment scales. Our goal was to determine whether the cognitively rehearsed, scripted response was effective in countering the stress effects of the uncivil encounter, and whether the response worked to the extent that work performance and patient safety were unaffected. Interestingly, though participants expressed confidence using cognitive rehearsal as an intervention prior to the simulation, responses indicated that a 60-minute session was insufficient to adequately prepare them to effectively address an uncivil encounter. For a detailed reporting of the findings, see Willhaus, Clark, and Kardong-Edgren (in review).

An Overview of Faculty-to-Faculty Incivility

One of the least studied areas of incivility in nursing education is the uncivil behavior experienced by faculty toward other faculty. We know that faculty conflicts, disagreements, and academic debates occur naturally within higher education and, if managed well, contribute to a robust intellectual learning environment (McElveen, Leslie, & Malotky, 2006).

However, if managed poorly or ignored, faculty discord can lead to faculty incivility and the disintegration of relationships. Some of the reasons given for faculty incivility include administrative inaction, a shift in culture from teaching to research with corresponding competition for scarce resources, and the emerging corporate culture of academia (Twale & De Luca, 2008).

While crafting the ANA position statement (ANA, 2015b) on workplace incivility, bullying, and violence, members of the panel decided to include information about mobbing because its impact can be devastating and lasting. Davenport, Schwartz, and Elliott (1999) defined *workplace mobbing* as "a malicious attempt to force out of the workplace through unjustifiable accusations, humiliation, general harassment, emotional abuse, and/or terror. It is a ganging up by the leader(s)— organization, superior, coworker, or subordinate who rallies others into systemic and frequent 'mob like' behavior. Because the organization ignores, condones, or even instigates the behavior, it can be said that the victim, seemingly helpless against the powerful and many, is indeed 'mobbed.' The result is always injury—physical or mental distress or illness and social misery and, most often, expulsion from the workplace" (p. 40).

Mobbing causes psychological, physical, social, and emotional damage and can have devastating economic consequences as the target fights to keep his or her job and career. The impact of mobbing is immeasurable, especially because in the early stages of mobbing or collective aggression, targets are often unaware that others have marked them for exclusion or expulsion from the group (Harper, 2013). If the mobbing behavior continues, targets may lose more than their perspective; in fact, the outcomes may be more devastating, including loss of one's reputation, professional identity, position, and economic livelihood.

In some cases, targets of mobbing may be outstanding employees or top performers ostracized for their exceptional contributions. Westhues (2004) suggested that mobbing among faculty members in academic workplaces may be related to envy of excellence and to jealousy associated with the achievements of others, including academic administrators' envy of faculty subordinates' excellence and high performance. A faculty participant in Heinrich's research (2007) related "joy-stealing" to an administrator's jealousy. Heinrich (2006a, 2006b) described 10 "joy-stealing games" that emerged from participants' stories of times they felt disrespected, devalued, and dismissed by faculty, staff, and administrative colleagues. Such behaviors poison interactions and contaminate collaborations, which can lead to an antagonistic, divided, and fragmented work environment (Heinrich, 2011). The author further noted that exclusion, competitiveness, envy, and lack of support might, in turn, impede and inhibit the advancement of faculty scholarship and research collaboration. Furthermore, the toxicity of these joy-stealing games can exert a detrimental effect on nurses' ability to contribute to the advancement of the knowledge base beyond the profession (Heinrich, 2011).

In 2013, I conducted a mixed-methodological study to build on Heinrich's work and to further understand the myriad dimensions of faculty-to-faculty incivility (Clark, 2013; Clark, Olender, Kenski, & Cardoni, 2013). The first part of the study was the quantitative portion and consisted of 588 nursing faculty representing 40 states in the United States. Faculty-to-faculty incivility was perceived as a moderate to serious problem. The behaviors reported to be most uncivil included faculty setting a coworker up to fail, making rude remarks or put-downs, and making personal attacks or threatening comments. The most frequently occurring incivilities included faculty members resisting change, failing to perform their share of the workload, distracting others by using media devices during meetings, refusing to communicate on work-related issues, and making rude comments or put-downs. The study found stress and demanding workloads to be two of the factors most likely to contribute to faculty-to-faculty incivility. Faculty reported fear of retaliation, lack of administrative support, and lack of clear policies as the top reasons for avoiding dealing with the problem of incivility.

The qualitative portion of the study asked faculty members to write a narrative account about an uncivil encounter they experienced with another faculty member and then to suggest the most effective ways to address faculty-to-faculty incivility. Some of the top themes in the narratives included faculty berating and insulting one another (often in faculty meetings), demeaning and belittling others, setting others up to fail, gossiping and spreading rumors, eye-rolling and other types of nonverbal disapproval, and taking credit for (ripping off) others' work and scholarly activities.

As I read the descriptions of faculty-to-faculty incivility and analyzed the findings, I was repeatedly struck by the destructive nature of uncivil faculty interactions. The stories were often related in the context of what I call the "in-group" and the "out-group" of nursing faculty teams (and I use the word *team* lightly). To illustrate this point, I want you to consider the following quotes taken from those stories:

> *We were attending a graduate faculty meeting when a member of the PhD faculty team rudely interrupted a DNP faculty member while she was presenting rationale for retaining a specific specialty track in the curriculum. The PhD member interrupted with a dismissive (snorting) noise and said, "This is a waste of my time. Everybody knows that [the specialty] isn't 'real' nursing. And anyway, the DNP isn't a 'real' doctorate, so I don't know why we should be discussing it at all."*

> *I met with my dean to seek advice about returning to graduate school to complete a doctoral degree—the dean laughed and said, "Are you kidding, at your age? You can't be serious. By the time you finish your degree, you'll be ready to retire. We prefer to invest in younger faculty."*

> *I am a member of the clinical faculty, and I can tell you unequivocally that we are a marginalized group. We are not considered part of the "real faculty" and are often referred to as "minions and underlings." We are frequently told that we have no clout, nor can we provide input into the theoretical courses or exams. And I just take it—it's like swallowing a very bitter pill.*

Not surprisingly, many of the stories contained feelings of rejection, dismissal, abuse, and marginalization. I found it very clear that we have a lot of work to do in nursing education to heal from these conditions and to build a culture of civility and collegiality. The majority of faculty suggested that we needed a direct approach to effectively communicate with one another. However, most respondents stated that they felt ill-equipped to deal with incivility. Many respondents requested faculty development workshops and sessions with experts brought in to help faculty learn to communicate effectively, constructively negotiate conflict, and to build a lasting culture of civility. Respondents also called for:

- Identifying skilled and effective leadership
- Eliminating power imbalances
- Hiring for civility and linking civility to job performance
- Empirically measuring the problem and implementing evidence-based solutions
- Developing and implementing policies, procedures, and guidelines
- Transforming the organizational culture
- Investing in relationship building through mentoring, scholarly collaborations, and celebrating accomplishments and achievements

An Overview of Student-to-Student Incivility

I have long been intrigued with the perceived state of student-to-student incivility in nursing education. In 2010, I conducted a qualitative study to gain a deeper understanding of this phenomenon. Fifty-three students responded to the survey. Thirty-one students reported an uncivil student encounter (58.4%) and provided a detailed description of the experience, and 41.6% stated that they had not experienced an uncivil student-to-student encounter.

Episodes of student-to-student incivility fell into six major categories:

- Making rude, sarcastic comments or verbal attacks
- Undermining and acting superior to other students
- Causing in-class disruptions
- Gossiping
- Dominating clinical time
- Making false accusations

When asked about their reactions or responses to the uncivil encounters, the majority of students avoided or ignored the encounter, politely addressed the behavior, or retaliated in kind. In response to the encounter, most respondents reported feeling angry, sad, or worried, or became ill in the aftermath of the encounter. In two cases, students thought poorly of the program for allowing students of such "poor quality" to be allowed entry into the nursing program. Most students coped with the effects of incivility by drawing on their inner strength, forgiving the person and "letting it go," or seeking encouragement from classmates or supportive faculty.

Following that initial study, I conducted a prospective mixed methodological longitudinal study (Clark, Nguyen, & Barbosa-Leiker, 2014). I followed one cohort of nursing students over a 3-year period to measure the group's perspectives of academic incivility, major stressors, most effective coping strategies, ways to improve student-to-faculty and student-to-student relationships, and advice to improve civility in the nursing program. I collected the data upon entry into the nursing program, 12 months into the nursing program, and at the end of the nursing program.

Perceived levels of civility declined slightly over the course of the 3-year study. The top two stressors remained constant through all three measurements: demanding workload and balancing work, school, family, and personal lives. However, the third stressor changed over time to include challenging clinical assignments and preparing for licensing exams. Most students coped by relaxing and spending time with others, exercising, and getting organized. Student-faculty relationships were enhanced by faculty presence and responsiveness, while student-to-student relationships were improved by supporting and encouraging one another. The most effective ways to foster civility included faculty encouragement, flexibility, and course organization and clarity.

My research clearly showed that raising awareness about the stressors of nursing education experienced by students and knowing the most effective coping strategies and ways to promote civility can have a major impact on improving the teaching-learning environment, building positive relationships among faculty and students, and addressing the challenges of academic incivility.

A Brief Overview of Incivility in the Online Learning Environment

According to the Association of International Educators (2010), the demand for higher education will double to approximately 200 million students by 2025, and much of this education will be delivered through distance and online learning programs. According to Bichsel (2013), nearly all institutions of higher learning in the United States (98%) have at least some departments, units, or programs with a major interest in e-learning, and many cite institutional advantages such as expanding enrollment, increasing revenue, enhancing their reputation, and streamlining curricula. The adoption of e-learning will also result in new business models for higher education, the need for student and faculty development, and the need to institute ways to maintain quality standards and, most importantly, to achieve student learning outcomes for a diverse group of learners. In recent years, the appeal of online learning has increased dramatically among students pursuing a degree in nursing and other health professions.

Earlier in this chapter I mentioned the work of Rieck and Crouch (2007), who discussed "connectivity" in the online learning environment in nursing courses and provided strategies to promote cybercivility. I have been interested in learning more about incivility in the online learning environment (OLE) for years. However, when I set out to examine this phenomenon in 2012, I quickly realized that I would need to create and psychometrically analyze an empirical instrument to measure the problem, especially because no tools existed to measure both faculty and student perspectives. The result was the creation of the Incivility in Online Learning Environment (IOLE) Survey, which was pilot tested and eventually used to conduct a mixed methodological study in a school of nursing. The two-part study was published later that year (Clark, Ahten, & Werth, 2012; Clark, Werth, & Ahten, 2012) and provided much-needed insight into faculty's and students' perceptions of and frequency of incivility in the OLE. The study also provided evidence-based strategies to prevent and address online incivility.

Participants in the study included 19 nursing faculty and 152 students enrolled in an online nursing course. Faculty respondents found incivility in the OLE to be a mild (38.9%) to moderate (38.9%) problem, whereas students found incivility in the OLE to be a mild (44.5%) to moderate (6.6%) problem. We also found that:

- 18.6% (faculty 16.7%; students 20.4%) of students and faculty were likely to engage in uncivil behavior

- 29% (faculty 38.9%; students 19.0%) perceived students as much more likely to engage in uncivil behavior in the OLE than in person

- Students are more likely than faculty to report cyberincivility

The uncivil student behaviors most frequently reported by students and faculty were identical and included failing to complete assignments in a timely manner; posting short, terse responses that did not add meaning to the online discussion; posting ambiguous or vague responses that did not add meaning to the online discussion; and failing to fulfill group responsibilities.

The uncivil faculty behaviors reported most frequently by faculty included having unclear expectations about assignments, failing to respond to students' postings in a timely manner, failing to post grades in a timely manner, and giving all students in a group the same grade regardless of effort or contribution. The uncivil faculty behaviors reported most frequently by students included having unclear expectations about assignments, posting a vague or confusing syllabus, failing to respond to student postings in a timely manner, assigning grades without providing useful feedback, and failing to post grades in a timely manner.

In the qualitative portion of the study, faculty and students reported several challenges associated with online learning. For example, faculty identified the very time-consuming tasks of reading, writing, and responding to student postings and assignments; the difficulty of attempting to create a sense of community and support in the OLE; and a lack of face-to-face contact. Students identified challenges of excessive group work, lack of faculty clarity and objectivity, and difficulty with being self-disciplined and on task in the OLE.

Both faculty and students identified flexibility, convenience, and the self-paced nature of the OLE as advantages. Faculty identified three strategies that students also identified to create civility in the

OLE: providing clearly defined course and behavioral expectations, norms, and consequences for uncivil behavior; faculty role-modeling of professionalism and civility; and addressing incivility immediately and holding offenders accountable. Unique items mentioned only by faculty included having faculty and students sign a civility statement and encouraging and rewarding civility; whereas items unique to the students were positive student role-modeling, providing civility orientation for all students, judicious or no use of group assignments, and increasing faculty responsiveness and availability.

De Gagne, Choi, Ledbetter, Kang, and Clark (2016), using the PRISMA (Preferred Reporting Items for Systematic Reviews and Meta-Analysis) framework, conducted an extensive literature review regarding cyberincivility in the health-related disciplines of medicine, nursing, and allied health. The intent of the review was to determine the extent to which health professional students and faculty experience cyberincivility, the direct and indirect effects and actions taken following cyberincivility, and ways to create and sustain civility and online learning environments. The authors suggested the development of clear policies related to online communication, development and implementation of policies related to its consequences, and formulation of guidelines for both student and faculty behavior online. The authors defined cyberincivility as "using communication technology to harass, intimidate, threaten, or otherwise harm others" (Hinduja & Patchin, 2010, p. 21) that can bring about deep emotional, physical, and social implications for everyone involved (Wankel & Wankel, 2012). The creation and maintenance of a safe, civil learning environment is particularly important because incivility is likely to interfere with the educator's ability to effectively teach and the student's ability to effectively learn. The topic of incivility in the OLE will be detailed further in Chapter 10.

Finishing Touches

The body of knowledge and science is growing regarding the myriad aspects of civility and incivility in nursing education—and that is definitely a good thing. We need to continue to study these issues and implement the best practices and strategies to prevent, address, and minimize the problem—and would it not be amazing if we could eradicate it altogether? Clearly, many other researchers have written other excellent papers that I have not summarized in this chapter, so I encourage you to read widely and deeply to seek and understand and then take bold and decisive action to be part of the civility solution.

CIVILITY TIP

Read deeply and broadly to familiarize yourself with the growing body of research on fostering civility in nursing education. Remember that you can make a significant individual and collective "civility" difference by measuring, addressing, and implementing evidence-based strategies to foster civility in all nursing organizations and settings.

Chapter 5

Raising Awareness, Naming the Problem, and Creating a Vision for Civility

It's too much to expect in an academic setting that we should all agree, but it's not too much to expect discipline and unvarying civility.
–John Howard, Australian statesman

This chapter discusses:

- Creating a healthy workplace
- Fashioning an organizational vision
- Assessing your civility competence

Creating Healthy Workplaces

Civility does not mean we all agree. In fact, faculty in higher education have a responsibility to create teaching-learning environments where lively debates and spirited discussions flourish. Our job is to foster social discourse, to question, and to pose critical arguments. Yet, to do this effectively, we must create safe spaces for all members of the campus community to express their views and beliefs. As ambassadors of the academy and gatekeepers to the profession, we must ensure civility is present in nursing education so that all members of the campus community benefit and thrive. Incivility is the kiss of death in any organization, and organizations must take steps to prevent and eradicate the problem. To do this, we must openly, courageously, and boldly address the problem—to name it and to encourage shared responsibility (faculty, students, administrators, and practice partners) to effectively address the problem. The end goal is to create and sustain a safe, healthy, and thriving teaching-learning environment where the organizational vision, mission, and values are shared, lived, and based on civility and respect.

All of us desire and deserve a workplace where we are valued, viewed as partners, and fairly rewarded for our contributions to the success of the organization. Highly desirable workplaces generate high levels of employee satisfaction, engagement, and morale, and encourage free expression of diverse ideas. The American Psychological Association (APA) recognizes psychologically healthy workplaces for their efforts to foster employee well-being while enhancing organizational performance (APA, 2015). According to the APA, healthy workplaces benefit from improved work quality and productivity, lower absenteeism, employee engagement, less turnover, and better customer service ratings.

Cockerell (2008) suggested that healthy workplaces are inclusive places, where all employees matter, are truly respected, valued, involved, and treated with dignity. The result of a healthy, inclusive workplace is one where employees are eager to come to work, ready to give their best, fully committed, creative, and loyal. Alternatively, when people do not feel included, they become apathetic and fail to perform at their full capacity. Inclusive workplaces are also reliant on strong and effective leaders who are readily available; communicate clearly, directly, and honestly; and role-model the behaviors they value and expect from others.

The Chronicle of Higher Education (2015) recognizes 13 categories of workplace excellence for institutions of higher education: collaborative governance, compensation and benefits, confidence in senior leadership, diversity, facilities, workspace and security, job satisfaction, professional/career development, respect and appreciation, supervisor or department chair relationship, teaching environment, tenure clarity in process, and work/life balance. Each year these criteria are used to identify colleges and universities determined by faculty, staff, and college administrators to be great places to work.

According to the American Nurses Association (ANA), a healthy work environment is one that is safe, empowering, and satisfying, and where all leaders, managers, healthcare workers, and ancillary staff perform with a sense of professionalism, accountability, transparency, involvement, efficiency, and effectiveness while being mindful of the health and safety of all persons (ANA, 2016). The recently revised edition of the American Association of Critical-Care Nurses' *Standards for Establishing and Sustaining Healthy Work Environments* reported that unhealthy work environments and relationship issues "can become the root cause of medical errors, hospital-acquired infections, clinical complications, patient readmissions, and nurse turnover" (AACN, 2016, p. 8). The AACN reaffirmed six standards for establishing and sustaining healthy work environments: skilled communication, true collaboration, effective decision-making, appropriate staffing, meaningful recognition, and authentic leadership.

In academia, the National League for Nursing (NLN) defined a healthful work environment in nursing education and published the Healthful Work Environment Tool Kit to assess nine elements (see the accompanying sidebar) that constitute a healthy academic work environment (NLN, 2006a). The tool kit provides a measurement for academic workplace assessment and a platform for discussion of how nursing faculty and administrators can work together to enhance healthy nursing academic workplaces. For a detailed and excellent discussion of healthy academic workplaces, see Brady (2010).

NATIONAL LEAGUE FOR NURSING (NLN) NINE ELEMENTS OF A HEALTHFUL WORK ENVIRONMENT TOOL KIT

- *Salaries*
- *Benefits*
- *Workload*
- *Collegial environment*

continues

- *Role preparation and professional development*
- *Scholarship*
- *Institutional support*
- *Marketing and recognition*
- *Leadership*

National League for Nursing Healthful Work Environment Tool Kit (2006a)

http://www.nln.org/docs/default-source/professional-development-programs/healthful-work-environment-toolkit.pdf?sfvrsn=2

Healthy academic work environments do not occur by accident—creating and sustaining them requires intentional and purposeful focus. I have taken the liberty to slightly expand on the work of the NLN on healthy academic workplaces and weave them into the nine elements with an explicit pursuit of civil workplaces. In addition to the elements included in the tool kit, I have added three additional aspects of a healthy work environment:

1. Establishing and committing to a shared vision, mission, values, and team norms

2. Creating and sustaining a high level of individual, team, and organizational civility and morale

3. Engaging in effective communication and constructive conflict negotiation at all levels of the organization

Nursing programs need to align their prospective vision, mission, and values with the institution at large and with a deliberate focus on civility and respect. See Chapter 2 for an exemplar of a university mission statement, statement of civility, and shared values. These documents and statements should be freely distributed and shared with all faculty, staff, students, and administrators (and campus visitors) because all parties are responsible for fulfilling them.

Assessing Your Civility Competence—Taking a Look in the Mirror

Begin by thinking about the elements of a healthy academic workplace. After you have them in mind, consider the most exciting, invigorating, and fulfilling work experience in your nursing career. In Chapter 1, I relate a bit of my early clinical practice as a psychiatric nurse working with troubled adolescents. During that time, I had the immense pleasure and tremendous satisfaction of being part of a hotshot crew of mental-health professionals who really clicked, worked well together, and consistently had each other's backs. Our clinical supervisor at the time, a well-known and well-respected child and adolescent psychiatrist, would often say that this was our "golden moment"—describing the incredible joy and satisfaction of being part of a high-performance work team engaged in very challenging but rewarding and meaningful work. Today, when I reflect on that time of my working life, I reflect on how extraordinary and unforgettable (and zestful!) it was.

My friend and colleague Kathleen Heinrich defines a golden moment as "a zestful interaction that leaves those involved glowing with a sense of well-being" (Heinrich, 2010a, p. 327). She encourages us to reflect on a "golden moment" interaction so we can use it as a baseline to rate our zest quotient (ZQ) on a "zest-o-meter" ranging on a scale from 0–10 (see Figure 5.1). So think back to a time (or perhaps it's occurring in your current workplace) when being a member of your work team left you glowing. If it is truly a "golden moment" experience, your ZQ will be 10—or even higher! Golden moment experiences can last for a brief period of time or for the life of a job. After you have rated your golden moment ZQ on the zest-o-meter, consider your current work situation and replot your ZQ. If your ZQ is a score consistently less than 8 or 9, you might want to examine whether your current work setting is the right fit for you. Many years ago, I worked in an organization where my ZQ score was rated below 5 every single day. I enjoyed my teammates and the patients were great, but sadly, the administrative team was seriously flawed. One of my closest and most trusted colleagues and I tried unsuccessfully for more than 2 years to use empirical evidence and patient-satisfaction survey data to sway the tide of ineffective leadership and its negative impact on patient care. It was a futile attempt, and in the end, the level and depth of incivility and incompetence were more than we could bear. We both left the organization.

0=No Zest   10=Extreme Zest

FIGURE 5.1

Zest-o-meter (Heinrich, 2010a).

Unfortunately, our experience is not unique. I recently received a phone call from a nurse educator seeking my counsel related to the incivility she was experiencing in her school of nursing. She was tearful and very upset, because two of her colleagues started spiteful rumors and gossiped about her to other faculty and students, claiming that the award she received for "Excellence in Teaching" was a joke and undeserved. The caller expressed how deeply she cared about her students and how important being a skilled teacher was to her. I asked the caller how she was coping with the matter, and she said, "I avoid my colleagues, because I hope that my solid reputation will prevail. If I was a novice educator, I would probably quit—maybe I still will." Over and over again, we hear about employees leaving organizations because of being treated badly and believing that life will be better elsewhere. With the current state of faculty shortages, we must do better.

Unfortunately, many faculty, students, and administrators are unaware of how their behaviors affect others. I enjoyed reading the story related by Pearson and Porath (2009) about a CEO who vowed to change his uncivil behavior after receiving feedback on his evaluation that he had a dreadful habit of making destructive comments about his employees. To break the habit, he promised $10 to anyone who caught him bad-mouthing the staff. He thought he might need to appeal to employees to get their support, but he quickly discovered that they were more than happy to lend a hand. By noon the first day, the CEO was out $50. But the strategy worked—the next day, he spent only $30 and was down to $10 the day after that. Before you know it, he had broken his uncivil habit.

Like the CEO, I firmly believe that we all need to carefully assess our civility aptitude and awareness. To assist in this assessment, I have created the Clark Workplace Civility Index to appraise one's level of civility competence. Treating one another with civility and respect is fundamental to establishing and sustaining healthy workplaces and fostering interpersonal and intrapersonal relationships. Civility is also essential to the development and ongoing success of top-performing work teams and for the achievement of first-rate, highly effective organizations. Reflecting and thinking deeply about civil and respectful interactions with others and engaging in thoughtful self-reflection are important steps toward improving our competence as leaders, colleagues, and team members. Obtaining colleague and/or mentor feedback on your Clark Workplace Civility Index improves awareness and helps determine strengths and areas for improvement.

Completing the Clark Workplace Civility Index requires time, thoughtful reflection, and courage. To begin, dedicate sufficient time and space to complete the index, find a quiet place void of distractions, and carefully consider the behaviors listed below (see the accompanying sidebar). Carefully consider the behaviors listed in the index; then respond truthfully and candidly regarding the perceived frequency of each behavior by answering 1) never, 2) rarely, 3) sometimes, 4) usually, or 5) always. Circle a response for each behavior, and then add up the number of 1–5 responses to determine the overall civility score. Scores range from 20–100.

CLARK WORKPLACE CIVILITY INDEX

Ask yourself, how often do I:
(1) Never (2) Rarely (3) Sometimes (4) Usually (5) Always

Assume goodwill and think the best of others	1	2	3	4	5
Include and welcome new and current colleagues	1	2	3	4	5
Communicate respectfully (by email, telephone, face-to-face) and really listen	1	2	3	4	5
Avoid gossip and spreading rumors	1	2	3	4	5
Keep confidences and respect others' privacy	1	2	3	4	5
Encourage, support, and mentor others	1	2	3	4	5
Avoid abusing my position or authority	1	2	3	4	5
Use respectful language (no racial, ethnic, sexual, age, or religiously biased terms)	1	2	3	4	5
Attend meetings, arrive on time, participate, volunteer, and do my share	1	2	3	4	5
Avoid distracting others (misusing media, side conversations) during meetings	1	2	3	4	5
Avoid taking credit for another individual's or team's contributions	1	2	3	4	5
Acknowledge others and praise their work/contributions	1	2	3	4	5
Take personal responsibility and stand accountable for my actions	1	2	3	4	5
Speak directly to the person with whom I have an issue	1	2	3	4	5
Share pertinent or important information with others	1	2	3	4	5
Uphold the vision, mission, and values of my organization	1	2	3	4	5
Seek and encourage constructive feedback from others	1	2	3	4	5
Demonstrate approachability, flexibility, and openness to other points of view	1	2	3	4	5
Bring my "A" game and a strong work ethic to my workplace	1	2	3	4	5
Apologize and mean it when the situation calls for it	1	2	3	4	5

Scoring the Civility Index: Add up the number of 1–5 responses to determine your civility score

90–100—Very civil	60–69—Minimally civil
80–89—Civil	50–59—Uncivil
70–79—Moderately civil	Less than 50—Very uncivil

After you have completed the index, consider your "civility" score. Are you satisfied? Are there areas for improvement? When you are ready, share your responses with a mentor or colleague to compare his or her assessment of your civility competence index with yours. Are there similarities? Are there differences or gaps? Spend time in conversation to discuss ways to maintain the positive aspects of your "civility index" and identify strategies to address aspects of your assessment you want to improve. After you have set your goals, make a plan to meet with your colleague and/or mentor to review progress on your goals. If your colleague or mentor is agreeable, perhaps you can provide similar feedback regarding his/her "civility index." As I suggested in Chapter 3, find a meeting place where both parties feel comfortable—a place that is quiet, undisturbed, and free of interruptions. You might enjoy walking and talking together in a serene area near campus or meeting in a quiet place away from the frantic pace of the workplace.

I have also used the Clark Workplace Civility Index with students in the clinical portion of my nursing leadership course. At the beginning of the course, students are made aware that during weeks 9 or 10 of the 15-week semester, they will be asked to complete the index based on their perceptions of themselves, and based on their perceptions of one of their classmates. We discuss as a group whether the dyads will be randomly selected or purposefully selected by the students themselves. The goal of the assignment is to engage in a self-reflection exercise, then practice giving and receiving constructive feedback—an essential skill for all nurses who will be asked to provide peer feedback in their role as professional nurses. This exercise provides students with an opportunity to practice these important and essential skills. The students thoughtfully complete the index outside of class so that they have sufficient time to reflect and carefully assess their own as well as their classmate's civility index. Students also identify one area for growth/improvement as well as identifying areas of strength for themselves and their classmate.

Once the day arrives for students to participate in the activity, using a large classroom, I have the dyads arrange themselves strategically so that they can engage in conversation without being affected by other students in the class. There are typically 12 students enrolled in my nursing leadership clinical course, so there are six dyads that can be easily spaced out in a large classroom. My job is to circulate and coach students if coaching is needed. I am constantly amazed at how well students engage in and take this activity seriously. Here's my suggestion to faculty: If students are up to the challenge of giving and receiving feedback, perhaps faculty can do the same.

Raising Awareness With Faculty

Raising awareness about the existence and consequences of incivility is an important and necessary step in fostering civility in nursing education. This awareness includes defining, encouraging, modeling, and embedding respectful behaviors into our workplaces. When nursing faculty and administrators agree upon and unite behind common expectations for how we are treated and how we treat others, we have the ability to change the culture (Clark & Ahten, 2011b). Faculty meetings are excellent venues to raise awareness about incivility, to discuss acceptable and unacceptable behaviors, to establish norms of behavior, and to practice and role-play civil interactions. When faculty members collectively co-create norms for behavior, they are more likely to approve of and conform to these behaviors.

> **NOTE**
>
> *Some ideas for faculty role-playing include ways to effectively engage in difficult conversations, negotiate conflict, and give and receive feedback. These suggestions are detailed in Chapter 9.*

Organizations also need to establish, implement, and widely disseminate confidential, non-punitive policies and procedures for addressing incivility—this includes enforcing sanctions if indicated and, perhaps more importantly, providing rewards for civility and collegiality. Although positive motivators are preferred, the consequences for violating the agreed-upon norms must be clearly stated and enforced. Ignoring or failing to address the uncivil behavior damages the organization as much, if not more, than the incivility itself.

NOTE

I am often asked to provide a list of "civility" incentives to use in creating a civil work environment. Although it would make the process easier, the truth is there is no one-size-fits-all answer. As Ken Blanchard (1999) so astutely stated, "What motivates people is what motivates people" (p. 46). Thus, academic leaders must ask their employees what motivates them—what they view as a meaningful reward and incentive for high performance. The responses will be as numerous and varied as the individuals involved and are powerful tools for leaders looking to engage their faculty in fostering civility.

While incentives vary from individual to individual, and while it is important for leaders to ask employees what motivates them, here are a few low-cost, high-impact reward ideas to get you started.

- Greet others by name and smile.
- Say "thank you" often; praise on the spot, and in the presence of others.
- Leave an appreciation note on their car or post a thank you note on their door.
- Treat a colleague to lunch.
- Give lottery or movie tickets, or a coffee shop gift card.
- Have the entire team sign a framed certificate of appreciation.
- Write an official note to one's file.
- Send a note of recognition to their family.

Ridding workplaces of incivility begins with leadership at all levels of the organization. Because an organization reflects the beliefs, attitudes, and actions of its leaders, leadership for its part must make a deliberate and conscious decision to eliminate uncivil behaviors, co-create norms and expectations for schools and workplaces, and hold all participants—including themselves—accountable. Change can only occur following public recognition of what behavior must be changed. Griffin (2010) stated that nursing "cannot fix the problem until we put a name to it. Throughout history, nursing has condoned intimidating behavior that has now become an 'acculturated bad behavior' that we don't really talk about." Put another way, James Baldwin stated, "Not everything that is faced can be changed, but nothing can be changed until it is faced." The profound and far-reaching effects of uncivil experiences cannot be minimized or marginalized. Thus, we must name it (incivility), own it, and work collaboratively to eliminate it.

Raising Awareness With Students

Raising awareness with students about incivility and discussing student responsibilities for promoting civility in educational and practice settings are vital endeavors and cannot be underestimated. Students at the very beginning of their nursing career need to know what is expected of them regarding professional behavior and what they can expect from others. In time, today's graduating students will become charge nurses, nurse managers, and valuable bedside nurses who might not have a title but are recognized as leaders among their peers. Students and new nurses will benefit most directly from education and policies in school and the workplace that clearly define expected professional academic and workplace behaviors, the process for addressing violations of those policies, and the consequences of those violations (Clark & Ahten, 2011b).

Institutions have several ways to raise awareness about incivility and its consequences with students but also, more importantly, to help them understand what civil, respectful, and professional behavior is; how to promote it and how to integrate civility into their daily lives. I suggest incorporating "civility" information explicitly into the agenda for incoming students during general student orientation. Nearly every college and university conducts an orientation for incoming students where they are introduced to a number of key topics to learn more about the institution, their role in its success, and ways to thrive in their academic pursuits. In our institution, I have been present during new student orientation and experienced firsthand how statements of civility and Shared Values are woven into the fabric of student orientation. Students learn what it means to be a member of the campus community, why civility matters, and how shared values provide a touchstone for all members of the campus community. From the very beginning, students entering the university understand the importance of civility and treating one another with mutual regard.

It would be great if all students attended new student orientation to the college/university; however, we know that is not the reality. In either case, orientation for new students enrolled in nursing programs needs to be carefully designed and intentional. The number of days dedicated to new student orientation varies; however, 3 days is recommended to allow sufficient time to engage students in interactive and collaborative learning activities to emphasize the key concepts of civility, professionalism, ethical practice, and socialization in the nursing profession (Clark, 2017). Prior to the on-campus orientation experience, online modules may be used to accomplish basic orientation needs such as securing health records and distributing the student handbook, policies, and procedures. Additionally, pre-assigned readings related to civility, professionalism, and ethical practice may be completed by students in advance of group activities conducted during on-campus orientation. The goal is to allow as much time as possible for other orientation activities conducted during on-campus orientation. These essential concepts are requisite to the delivery of safe, quality, patient-centered care.

Active learning exercises can be incorporated to highlight specific evidence and rationale for fostering civility leading to safe patient care. Some examples include discussion of High Reliability Organizations (HROs), the ANA *Code of Ethics* (2015a), Institute of Medicine *Future of Nursing* report (2011), ANA *Scope and Standards of Practice* (2015c), and Quality and Safety Education for Nurses (QSEN, 2016) competencies. Other activities for learner engagement during new student orientation include "slicing the civility pie" and incorporating freewrites focused on the students' responsibility in fostering civility, professionalism, and ethical practice (Clark, 2017).

Some nursing programs across the United States are including formal White Coat Ceremonies as part of their orientation experience. They are commonly held upon entry into the nursing program and symbolize a professional rite of passage to welcome students into the profession. The ceremonies typically include a keynote address delivered by a nurse leader and marked by students taking a public oath acknowledging their commitment to the profession. The ceremony is commemorated by the donning of the white coat and/or a lapel pin as visual evidence of the students' commitment to quality patient care (Clark, 2017).

In my faculty role, I commonly facilitated sessions during new student orientation and throughout the nursing students' progression through the program. The concepts of civility, professionalism, and ethical practice are explicitly discussed, and active learning strategies are implemented to bring the content to life. While it was my responsibility to facilitate much of the civility conversation during new student orientation and beyond, it is important for all faculty and administrators in the school of nursing to reinforce and extend the message in a variety of interesting and creative ways. In the initial orientation class, I present an overview of the state of the science on civility and incivility in nursing education and practice, discuss how the vision and shared values of the school of nursing provide a foundation for civility, and engage students in activities focused on what they can do to promote respectful interactions throughout their nursing program. One of my favorite activities is to have students participate in slicing the "civility pie." I provide the students with a large index card that is blank on both sides. Working independently, I ask each student to draw a large circle on one side of the index card—and this is that person's "civility pie." Then, I ask each student to consider how much of the pie students, faculty, and school administrators are responsible for in promoting civility and to slice the pie accordingly. After students divide their pies, I ask them to turn their cards over and provide a rationale for why they sliced their pies the way they did. I then ask the students to assemble into small groups (learning circles) to discuss their individual responses—and to share their rationale for why they cut the pie the way they did. Then, I ask students to select one example (or to create a new one) based on their small-group discussions. Once the students select a pie and rationale, I ask them to take a picture on their smartphone and email it to me so that I can randomly select three or four civility pies and rationales to project on a display screen so that they can be discussed in a large-group session. This exercise can be modified to fit the individual needs of the class and faculty preference.

Since starting this exercise several years ago, I have had nearly 80% of students divide their pies into thirds, indicating that each group is equally responsible for fostering civility. Other students have sliced the pie in various ways; my favorite "slice" is when students draw three circles around the perimeter of the pie, stating that all three groups (students, faculty, and administrators) are 100% responsible for fostering civility. Brilliant!

Over the years, students have provided interesting rationales regarding the importance of fostering civility and expressing why they sliced their civility pie the way they did (see the accompanying sidebar). This is a wonderful exercise to do with students and provides a useful platform to identify and discuss specific ways for students to promote civility throughout their nursing programs and beyond.

STUDENT RATIONALE FOR SLICING THE CIVILITY PIE

Each of us should be accountable for 100% of the civility pie. That way, we take responsibility for our own actions and set a professional example.

I believe students, faculty, and administration have/share equal parts in creating an environment of civility. It's a shared responsibility for everyone no matter what "role" you play!

Everyone has the responsibility to show respect to each other. Treat others the way you want to be treated...it doesn't matter whether you are a student or a teacher. Everyone deserves to have respect and show respect to others.

A group is a representation of its leadership. Faculty and students look toward administrators to set an example of acceptable characteristics; therefore, 50% of the civility pie belongs to administration.

After we have discussed civility and incivility and shared our civility pie and rationale, I put a PowerPoint slide up on the screen. The slide is titled, "How Can Students Promote Civility?" A student volunteer types student responses into the slide while I facilitate class discussion on specific ways that students can foster civility. The box on the next page depicts the suggestions identified in one of my orientation classes.

HOW CAN STUDENTS PROMOTE CIVILITY (DR. CLARK'S STUDENT ORIENTATION)

Respect others and follow the Golden Rule.

Assume goodwill and think the best of others.

Be honest and nonjudgmental.

Be inclusive and collaborative.

Use open and respectful communication.

Be humble and fair.

Stand for something good.

Don't personalize, let things go—and show forgiveness.

Another engaging civility activity is to have students complete the Clark Civility Index for Students and Classmates (see sidebar). Similar to the Clark Workplace Civility Index shown earlier in this chapter, the index for students is designed to raise awareness, measure perceptions of civility acumen, generate discussion, and provide a mechanism for giving and receiving constructive feedback. The index can be used in a number of ways. One way is to provide the students with an exact copy of the index printed on each side of a piece of paper. In most cases, I do not ask for any identifying information (that is, name, class, etc.) because I am more interested in receiving candid, honest responses. Using the front side of the paper, students are asked to complete the index based on their perceptions of themselves; then, on the other side of the paper, students complete the index again based on their perceptions of their classmates. After discussing what it was like to complete the index and sharing insights, I collect the completed indices and summarize the results so that I can share them with students during a subsequent class session. The results make for interesting conversation, because in nearly every case, students rate themselves higher on the civility index than they rate their classmates. Chapter 9 includes the Clark Civility Index for Faculty.

CLARK CIVILITY INDEX FOR STUDENTS & CLASSMATES

To complete the index, consider the 20 statements listed below. Read each statement carefully and select the response that most accurately represents the frequency of each behavior.

Ask yourself, how often do I:
(1) Never (2) Rarely (3) Sometimes (4) Usually (5) Always

Role-model civility, professionalism, and respectful discourse	1	2	3	4	5
Add value and meaning to the educational experience	1	2	3	4	5
Communicate respectfully (by email, telephone, face-to-face) and really listen	1	2	3	4	5
Avoid gossip and spreading rumors	1	2	3	4	5
Avoid making sarcastic remarks or gestures (staged yawning, eye-rolling)	1	2	3	4	5
Pay attention and participate in class discussion and activities	1	2	3	4	5
Use respectful language (avoid racial, ethnic, sexual, gender, religiously biased terms)	1	2	3	4	5
Avoid distracting others (misusing media, devices, side conversations) during class	1	2	3	4	5
Avoid taking credit for someone else's work or contributions	1	2	3	4	5
Co-create and abide by classroom and clinical norms	1	2	3	4	5
Address disruptive student behaviors and promote a safe, civil learning environment	1	2	3	4	5
Take personal responsibility and stand accountable for my actions	1	2	3	4	5
Speak directly to the person with whom I have an issue	1	2	3	4	5
Complete my assignments on time and do my share of the work	1	2	3	4	5
Arrive to class on time and stay for the duration	1	2	3	4	5
Avoid demanding make-up exams, extensions, grade changes, or other special favors	1	2	3	4	5
Uphold the vision, mission, and values of my organization	1	2	3	4	5
Listen to and seek constructive feedback from others	1	2	3	4	5
Demonstrate an openness to other points of view	1	2	3	4	5
Apologize and mean it when the situation calls for it	1	2	3	4	5

Scoring the Civility Index: Add up the number of 1–5 responses to determine your civility score

90–100—Very civil	60–69—Minimally civil
80–89—Civil	50–59—Uncivil
70–79—Moderately civil	Less than 50—Very uncivil

We also discuss additional ways that students can promote civility, including engaging in stress-reducing behaviors and assuming personal responsibility to co-create classroom and clinical norms and to conform and abide by them. We discuss the importance of modeling civility; engaging in respectful social discourse; and participating on teams, committees, and governance councils. We also reinforce the significance of attending class, being on time, being prepared, avoiding side conversations, and not using media in disruptive ways. This is just the beginning of the activities that occur across the curriculum. Faculty and students collaborate to co-create classroom norms, to foster a safe teaching-learning environment, and consistently discuss the imperative of civility in nursing education and practice.

Creating an Organizational Vision for Civility

A clear organizational vision helps everyone understand what the organization is trying to achieve, assists in overcoming forces that hinder progress, and clearly articulates a collective sense of what a desirable future looks like. Organizations everywhere are undergoing significant change, and nursing education is no exception. Nursing programs face several challenges, including pressure to manage costs while maintaining or improving student admission and retention rates, National Council Licensure Examination (NCLEX) scores, and faculty recruitment and retention rates; identifying opportunities for growth; dealing with financial uncertainty; and stewarding limited resources. Thus, nurse leaders, educators, and students must work together to create and sustain a safe, civil academic environment. For some programs, this is a daunting task requiring time, resources, leadership, and commitment to long-term change. Transforming the culture also requires changing the conversation, revising our assumptions about people, respecting one another's point of view, and creating a meaningful vision of the future (Showkeir & Showkeir, 2008).

Leaders play a key role in defining the future, aligning people with a compelling vision, and inspiring action to achieve the new vision. Creating and reaching agreement on a shared vision takes time, continual communication, and an ardent commitment to long-term cultural change. Organizations can choose from various frameworks for developing an organizational vision, but Latham (1995) is my favorite (see the nearby sidebar). The framework provides a clear, systematic structure for creating a collective and shared vision of the future. The eight steps to Latham's framework are summarized in the paragraphs that follow.

To be successful, a vision should represent the values and principles of the organization at large. A "vision" team of five to seven trusted and credible individuals from throughout the organization might be well-suited to draft and create the vision. The team should collect broad-based input by asking people their opinions about an ideal organizational culture, ways to promote personal and professional development, services to be offered, and ways to promote excellence and recognition for all members of the organization. After this information is collected, the team can begin brainstorming. Brainstorming is an effective way to generate divergent ideas and a valuable tool to stimulate creative thinking. Members of the vision team can ask themselves the same survey questions to help visualize and develop a vivid picture of a great organization.

After information is gathered from members of the organization, the vision team must "shrink the mess" by reducing the large number of ideas generated by the group down to a smaller, more manageable number without losing content. This can be accomplished by eliminating duplication, deleting any suggestions or ideas that are inappropriate or clearly do not fit, and then categorizing the main ideas into themes. Next, the vision team creates a rough draft of the vision statement to create a vivid representation of the organization's future—a very important step that requires considerable time and attention. Before taking the vision to the organization for approval, the team considers whether the vision statement is timeless, is inspirational, and provides decision-making criteria. If it passes this test, it is ready to be vetted by the organization. The vision statement is presented to the entire organization for approval. The team needs to explain the process it went through to create the vision and to clarify the vision statement, and the team must be open to modifications. The final step in the process is a refinement of a clear, well-developed, shared vision statement that expresses a clear purpose, directs strategic initiatives, and enables the organization to maintain constancy of purpose.

DEVELOPING AN ORGANIZATIONAL VISION (LATHAM, 1995)

1. *Collect input.*
2. *Brainstorm.*
3. *Shrink the mess.*
4. *Develop the rough draft.*
5. *Refine the statement.*
6. *Test the criteria.*
7. *Obtain approval.*
8. *Communicate and celebrate.*

After the vision is firmly established, it must be communicated frequently, broadly, and convincingly. We must discuss it and share it in hallways, break rooms, classrooms, and clinical settings. Collectively, we must keep our "eye on the ball" and continually focus on the desired vision and strategic steps to achieve it. As soon as we are living and fulfilling our shared vision, we must anchor it in the culture by deeply embedding civility and teamwork in that culture, adopting a statement of shared values and guiding principles, having a working set of cultural norms, and implementing effective policies and procedures to support the new vision. Successful and lasting change of an organization's culture can take years and begins with an inspirational and compelling vision for change and transformation.

Finishing Touches

Raising awareness about the problem of rude and disruptive behavior and uncovering the serious and insidious nature of incivility go a long way in eliminating it from workplaces and other organizations. When we stand together and amplify the local and national dialogue of promoting civility, it sends a powerful message that cannot be ignored. Taking a careful personal inventory of our own civility competence and creating clear, purposeful organizational visions that reflect a true commitment to civility and mutual respect provide firm foundations for creating and sustaining civil work environments.

CIVILITY TIP

Be courageous, and with absolute candor, complete the Workplace Civility Index by assessing your own level of civility competence. Invite a trusted colleague to do the same, and then make a date to exchange your assessments. Make a plan to improve in at least one area, and keep doing the behaviors that make your civility competence soar.

Chapter 6
Principled Leadership and the Power of Positive Role-Modeling and Mentoring

If your actions inspire others to dream more, learn more, do more and become more, you are a leader.
–John Quincy Adams

This chapter discusses:

- Defining principled leadership
- Crafting a personal, professional vision of the future
- Positive role-modeling and mentoring

The Power and Influence of Principled Leadership

Leaders in nursing education (or in any organization, for that matter) exist at every level of the organization—some hold formal positions with titles, whereas others have informal positions and no title. Formal leaders hold a position of authority and an assigned role within the organization that involves a span of influence. Informal leaders, on the other hand, hold no formal title or authority but are advocates for the organization and heighten productivity through influence, relationship-building, knowledge, and expertise. In any case, "real" leaders make a significant contribution to the organization and to the development of themselves and others as leaders and are nimble enough to adapt, change, and add value to the organization and to the people it serves. As Kouzes and Posner (2012) clearly remind us, the best organizations are those where everyone, regardless of title or position, is encouraged to act like a leader and is rewarded for doing so. According to the authors, the top four most important leadership characteristics include being honest, forward-looking, competent, and inspiring. These desired leadership attributes "have remained constant in the ever-changing and turbulent social, political, and economic environment of the past 30 years" (Kouzes & Posner, 2012, p. 36).

According to Northouse (2012), leadership has both moral and ethical dimensions, primarily because leaders influence the lives of others. Leadership (whether formal or informal) carries an enormous ethical responsibility. Put simply, *ethical leadership* is the influence of a moral person who moves others to do the right thing, in the right way, for the right reasons (Ciulla, 2003). Northouse further notes that three main principles direct the actions of ethical leaders: showing respect, serving others, and showing justice (2012). Similarly, Yoder-Wise (2015) describes leadership as a willingness to identify and act on complex problems in an ethical manner; it is not coercive or manipulative, and an ethical leader keeps others informed and engages them in co-creating solutions to meet organizational needs. Ethical leaders are trustworthy; foster open-ended and meaningful conversation and critique; consider all aspects of an issue while searching for a non-adversarial, problem-solving outcome; are inclusive; and ultimately encourage honest and ethical behavior.

Honesty is a significant factor in our leaders—we want our leaders to be truthful, ethical, and principled. We want leaders with integrity with whom we can enjoy a dependable and trusting relationship. Warren Bennis (2009) reminds us that becoming a leader is similar to the process of becoming an integrated human being and that all successful leaders have certain characteristics in common—a clear vision, passion, and integrity. Bennis further describes the "Four Lessons of Self-Knowledge" needed to be a successful leader:

1. Being your own best teacher by engaging in continuous learning through personal transformation that occurs with each new lesson and challenge

2. Accepting responsibility and avoiding blame

3. Being a devoted and passionate learner

4. Self-reflecting to gain true understanding by reflecting on our experiences, discovering the truth about ourselves, and making meaning of the discovery

Figure 6.1 shows a model based on these four lessons.

FIGURE 6.1

Four lessons of self-knowledge for leaders (adapted from Bennis, 2009).

An organization needs the expertise and talents of many individuals and teams to realize the organizational vision. As such, each of us must make a commitment to pursue "personal mastery"—an ongoing commitment to unfolding and authentically expressing who we are (Cashman, 1998); appreciating the rich mixture of our life experiences, how they dynamically form our unique existence; and then integrating them into a meaningful context (Cashman, 2008). Exercising personal mastery is a lifelong development challenge that might best be accomplished by genuinely exploring our deeply held personal beliefs, because our beliefs create, influence, and provide a lens for interpreting our reality (Cashman, 2008). For example, if individuals believe it is acceptable behavior to disregard and diminish others, they are more likely to treat others with contempt. On the other hand, if treating others with respect and civility is important, then people will be more likely to take a positive view of others. Thus, examining our personal biases and beliefs helps us become more conscious and self-aware. This journey toward continuous individual improvement must be guided by a personal, professional vision, including the action steps to achieve it.

In Chapter 5, I discussed the process of developing a compelling and inspirational organizational vision. Here, I describe a similar process for developing our desired personal, professional vision of our future. The renowned futurist Joel Barker once said:

Vision without action is merely a dream

Action without vision just passes the time

Vision with action can change the world

I firmly believe that this is true. We must bolster our personal currency and strengthen our potential to do great things by defining our positive vision for the future. To contemplate our positive vision of our future, consider Viktor Frankl's riveting book *Man's Search for Meaning* (1959), which chronicles Frankl's grueling experience in a Nazi concentration camp during the Holocaust. Frankl's gripping account describes how the power of vision enabled prisoners to find a reason to live under the most deplorable and despicable conditions ever perpetrated on humanity. Frankl concluded that the meaning of life is found in every moment of living (as well as suffering) and that striving to find meaning in one's life is the primary motivational human force. Frankl writes, "It is a peculiarity of man that he can only live by looking to the future. And this is his salvation in the most difficult moments of his existence" (p. 81).

Crafting a meaningful personal, professional vision of our future requires thoughtful reflection and introspection. As Sullivan (2013) notes, "Visioning is the process of imagining our preferred future and deciding on the steps to make that future happen" (p. 82). It cannot be done instantaneously; it requires thinking, mulling over, and "time for incubation" (Sullivan, 2013, p. 83). Creating a personal, professional vision of our future involves asking ourselves some very important and probing questions.

First, we need to carefully identify (and ultimately commit to and live by) a set of unwavering principles, values, and daily habits. Clarifying our principles and values helps us become more self-aware, make ethically based decisions, set goals, prioritize roles and responsibilities, develop as a leader—and ultimately chart our personal, professional course for a positive future.

There are several excellent tools to clarify principles and values; my personal favorite is the Values Exercise by Kouzes and Posner (2012). This exercise can help us identify our principles and values; however, discussing and clarifying our principles and values with a trusted mentor is another great way to solidify our unshakable beliefs. From there we can determine and practice our daily habits. Whatever method you prefer to employ, it is absolutely essential that we be clear and mindful of the principles and values that guide our actions and daily habits. I have included my principles and daily habits in the sidebar nearby.

PRINCIPLES

- *Lead a purposeful and examined life*
- *Assume best intentions—fill the reservoir of goodwill*
- *Bask in the cathedral of the blue dome*
- *Nurture and exercise body, mind, and spirit every day*
- *Endorse the 3 R's (relationships, relationships, relationships)*

continues

continued

DAILY HABITS

- *Smile and greet others (by name when possible)*
- *Be a positive and intentional role model*
- *Enjoy the outdoors, breathe, and move*
- *Express gratitude—and count my blessings*
- *Act with kindness—pay compliments*
- *Make a difference and stand for something good*

Now, take a moment to consider the principles and values that shape your life. How might they form the foundation to craft your personal, professional vision of the future—and how do they influence your daily habits?

To craft your personal, professional vision of your future, consider your current reality (where you are today), your desired future (tomorrow), and the action steps you need to take to achieve your ideal vision (see Figure 6.2). The difference between our current and desired future reality is called "creative tension" (Senge, 1990)—the energy used to move us from where we are to where we want to be. Sometimes this tension creates anxiety, which, in this case, is a positive sign that we are giving due diligence to establishing our desired vision.

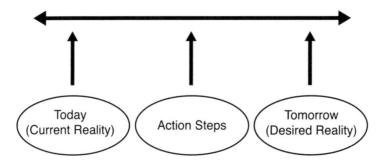

FIGURE 6.2

Crafting a personal, professional vision of the future.

Next, imagine yourself 3, 5, or 10 years from now, and answer this question: If you could create the career or the life of your dreams, what would it look like? Then, picture yourself a year before retirement—as you look back on your career, what will you wish you had done or accomplished? What is the legacy you want to leave? "Beginning with the end in mind" (Covey, 1989, p. 98) helps us imagine "the end" as a frame of reference by which everything else is examined and helps us start with a clear understanding of our destination. Covey believes that we cannot be effective unless we begin with the end in mind. That said, remember that things can and will change, so be flexible, and be ready to revise your vision when unplanned events occur, but stay focused on the prize (your vision).

Next, think about the action steps that will "get you there"—consider the following questions to guide you:

1. What am I doing today that will help me achieve my goals tomorrow?

2. How am I doing on focusing on the important things in my life?

3. How and where am I committing my time? Is this a sound investment?

4. What is my next step toward career success?

5. What parts of my life can I simplify—what can I say "no" to?

6. How will my plans affect my family and friends?

7. If I could change something in my life, what would it be?

8. Am I satisfied with the direction of my career/life?

9. What is missing in my career/life? How can I achieve what's missing?

10. Will my chosen profession get me up in the morning and bring me joy?

Another helpful exercise in creating our personal, professional vision of a desired future involves intentional and purposeful self-evaluation. To complete this exercise (Pisanos, 2011), find time for quiet reflection and contemplate the fill-in-the-blank questions in the accompanying sidebar.

REFLECTION AND SELF-EVALUATION (PISANOS, 2011)

Self

The part of myself I am willing to work on is _____

_____

The part of myself I celebrate is _____

_____

Others

An aspect of my relationships I am willing to improve is _____

_____

The ways I engage in relationships I celebrate are _____

Skills

The skill(s) I am willing to improve are _____

_____

The skills I celebrate in myself are _____

_____

Environment

The ways I am willing to engage differently in my workplace are

_____

I positively contribute to my workplace by _____

_____

Now that you have considered and imagined your desired future, what do you see? Is your vision concise and pithy enough to fit on a T-shirt or a coffee cup? For example, my vision reads, "Leading the coalition for change: Creating and sustaining communities of civility." How about your vision? Is it succinct enough to be stated in a single sentence? Does it include civility and respect? If not, you might want to revisit and revise your vision statement, because civility is fundamental to a successful and serene life (Forni, 2002). When you are satisfied with your vision statement, share it with others, discuss its meaning, and celebrate your future.

When I facilitate the visioning process with faculty and student groups, in general, they find the experience challenging, though fulfilling. I frequently share my personal, professional vision with others and include some of my "action steps," which consist of being an outspoken and ardent leader to create and sustain communities of civility, to inspire healthy workplaces and relationships, to amplify the national dialogue on fostering civil work and learning environments, and to be an ambassador for lasting change. I encourage faculty and students to be courageous and bold, and to ignore the naysayers who declare they cannot achieve their dreams. I challenge them (and all of us) to become passionate and enthusiastic *civility champions*—advocates for a more civil society. I inspire them to live by the principles of civility noted by Dr. Michael Woods (2010), who states that these principles are nearly identical to the principles of leadership. The six principles of civility include respect, empathy, flexibility, interest in other cultures, tolerance, and the acquisition and practice of technical skills (Cherlynn Conetsco, as cited in Woods, 2010, p. 9). I remind them to stay focused and true to their convictions—to visualize achieving their goals and celebrating each and every success toward accomplishing them. As the prominent comedian Joe E. Lewis stated, "You only live once—but if you work it right, once is enough."

The Imperative of Principled, Ethical, Authentic, Kind (PEAK) Leadership

From inspired works on skilled leadership and through our own experiences, we have learned that respected leaders are visionary, trustworthy, honest, fair, and inclusive. They exercise sound judgment, use science and evidence to make well-informed decisions, and are often described as prudent, generous, compassionate, and humble. They inspire *esprit de corps*, hope, teamwork, and collaboration. In my *Musing of the Great Blue* blog post (Clark, 2016) titled "The imperative of PEAK leadership," I assert unequivocally that character matters and that we should each aspire to be PEAK leaders—leaders who are *principled, ethical, authentic, and kind.*

Principled leaders utilize well-defined values and sound principles to guide decisions and to determine the clearest direction, especially during turbulent times. Principled leaders are continual learners, service-oriented, courageous, and synergistic. They are formidable role models who live by a well-reasoned personal philosophy and a firmly established set of values and beliefs that engender trust, respect, and inclusivity. Principled leaders are characterized by personal integrity, by respect for the rights and dignity of others, and by setting a positive example for all members of the organization.

Similar to principled leadership, ethical leaders are honest and embrace the belief that character is defined by the way we behave and treat others. They also lead by example, model the way, and recognize that respect must be given as well as earned. They focus on developing others, taking responsibility for their actions, and celebrating the successes of others. They do what is right rather than what is expedient, convenient, or self-serving. Ethical leaders communicate frequently and openly; they encourage expression of new ideas and alternate ways of doing things. They cultivate a positive work environment and hold themselves and others to a high standard of excellence and ethical conduct.

In a comparable fashion, authentic leaders are deeply committed to self-awareness, knowing and understanding one's strengths and areas for improvement, and reflecting upon who we are at our deepest level. Authentic leaders carefully examine their emotions, motives, goals, and core values—and inspire others to do the same. They are transparent, honest, and open—they are genuine, connected to other members of the organization, and consistently demonstrate character and integrity.

Kind leadership is synonymous with compassionate and generous leadership. Many leaders prefer to lead from their head and fail to acknowledge the power of leading from the heart. Unfortunately, many of today's workplaces are characterized by incivility and bullying, causing some non-PEAK leaders to take hard, directive, and sometimes abusive positions in order to force others to follow their command without question or recourse. Some believe that leading with kindness and compassion are signs of weakness. But, in reality, it is just the opposite. Leading with kindness and compassion is evidence of strength, courage, and mettle. Expressing kindness in the workplace and simply being mindful of the effect our words and actions have on others can be a real leadership advantage. Showing appreciation, finding opportunities to praise and acknowledge others, and extending a generous spirit are more likely to foster trust, increase employee engagement, and achieve organizational goals.

Positive Role-Modeling

I would like to begin this section with a quote from Rumi, a poet, scholar, theologian, and mystic, that speaks to the importance of positive role-modeling. Rumi states, "Yesterday I was clever so I wanted to change the world. Today I am wise, so I am changing myself." It takes courage and commitment to look in the mirror—and to make an honest appraisal of who we are and how we come across to others. In Chapter 5, I introduced readers to the Clark Workplace Civility Index as a tool to assess civility acumen and evaluate how we interact and relate with others. Kouzes and Posner (2012) clearly acknowledge that leadership is about relationships, credibility, and what we do and how we behave. Leadership requires us to look inward, to reflect, and to establish a clear set of principles and values by which to lead a purposeful and meaningful life.

Establishing an organizational Civility Code and a Statement of Shared Values (SSV) provides a foundation for desired individual and collective behavior, makes explicit what an institution stands for, and builds a sense of community (Connelly, 2009). Further, civility must be modeled in accordance with the SSV so that it becomes a lived reality. All members of the organization share the responsibility to be positive, ethical, and civil role models by demonstrating the behaviors and characteristics they wish to see. Leaders set the tone and must model respect for all individuals, including (and perhaps most importantly) for those who have an opposing point of view. Open social discourse can only take place in an environment built on trust and respect. We all have the potential and capacity to be powerful role models, and we consistently send messages and clues as to what we consider to be acceptable behavior. Even when we do not exhibit incivility, we, in essence, condone it if we ignore or fail to address it. Failing to take heed of and deal with uncivil behaviors damages the organization as much, if not more, than the incivility itself. In our school of nursing, our behavioral norms provide a framework for modeling civility not only for our students but for one another. We focus on assuming goodwill, showing inclusion and respect, being transparent and responsive, using direct communication, maintaining confidentiality, and following the Golden Rule—to do to others as you would have them do to you. Civil role models inspire us and are individuals we wish to emulate. In many cases, we are or can be the civil role models. Some of the common characteristics of civil role-modeling in the workplace are provided in the accompanying sidebar.

The National League for Nursing (NLN) *Core Competencies of Nurse Educators* (2005) requires nursing faculty to serves as role models for professional nursing. Positive faculty role-modeling is critical for student development and for socialization into the nursing profession. As faculty members become more focused on student "formation," role-modeling becomes even more important, because the formation process includes "shaping the habits and dispositions for use of knowledge and skilled-know-how [that] occurs in every aspect of a nursing student's education" (Benner, Sutphen, Leonard, & Day, 2010, p. 88). In other words, it is "impossible to predict what experiences will be pivotal for a student" (Benner et al., 2010, p. 89). Thus, modeling professional behavior, attire, language, and communication is critical to student learning and to future success in the practice setting (Clark, 2009). Effective communication can be modeled by using respectful language, maintaining inclusive attitudes, teaching and demonstrating civil discourse, and listening to and intentionally conversing with students.

COMMON CHARACTERISTICS OF CIVIL ROLE MODELS

Contemplative and humble

Respectful of colleagues

Catalysts for change and transformation

Facilitators and team players

Collegial and empowering of others

Trustworthy and honest

Effective communicators

Responsible, accountable, and willing to admit mistakes

Self-assured without being self-important

Engaged in self-care and healthy stress management

Another aspect of role-modeling requires faculty to be connected to the practice of nursing where our students learn and work. As nursing faculty, we must be current in clinical practices so that we can role-model and prepare our students to enter, navigate, and achieve success in the practice environment. Faculty (and peer) support fosters confidence and improves open communication (Del Prato, Bankert, Grust, & Joseph, 2011).

Finally, to be effective role models, faculty members must be aware of their own behavior. Some faculty members display uncivil behaviors by belittling or demeaning others, asserting their superiority, or excluding and marginalizing coworkers (Clark, 2008a; Clark, 2013). These and similar behaviors invite a reciprocal process of incivility in protest against perceived unfair or unreasonable treatment. Therefore, we must consistently examine our interactions, teaching methods, conduct, and communication styles. By doing so, we can avoid unnecessary conflict with others and foster collegial relationships. Modeling respectful treatment of others, expressing appreciation, and supporting one another cultivates a vibrant and fertile culture of civility where people enjoy working, learning, and growing.

Positive Mentoring: Celebrating Our Rock Stars and Rising Stars

If I have seen a little further it is by standing on the shoulders of giants.
–Sir Isaac Newton

Mentoring is a relationship between an individual with potential (*mentee*) and an individual with expertise (*mentor*). The role of the mentor is to guide the professional development of the mentee by sharing knowledge, experience, wisdom, and perspective within a context of mutual respect and trust. A true mentor advises and guides, encourages and serves as a role model, and offers honest criticism and informal feedback—all while establishing and maintaining professional boundaries and relationships. Mentors are generous, competent, confident; focus on mutual benefit; and possess a nurturing soul. Mentoring relationships are not confined by time and place; can occur at any point in one's career; are characterized by collegiality and collaboration; are not limited by age or experience;

and are centered on personal, professional growth. Mentees demonstrate initiative and curiosity, a desire to learn, a commitment to improvement, and a willingness to seek guidance.

As nurse educators, we are leaders and mentors and are called upon to mobilize purposeful, evidence-based, transformational change. Each of us needs not only to seek out strong and influential mentors to guide our own life and career but also to "pay it forward" by mentoring others.

My life has been enriched and enlightened by the formidable role models and mentors in my life. Early on, my mother and maternal grandmother reinforced the value of relationships and service to others. Later, when I entered the university and encountered various professors, several influenced my life in positive ways. Most prominent among them was a nursing professor I refer to as Professor Sweet (as I mentioned in Chapter 1) who inspired me to become the nurse and the person I am today. Many of us have achieved remarkable accomplishments in our lives and in our careers. For most, our dreams and achievements are largely realized because of the incredible mentors and nursing "giants" that have encouraged and supported us along our nursing and life's journey— strong, impressive mentors who have paved the way and illuminated the path to excellence. I would like to share a personal story of one of my own mentoring experiences that helped launch my nursing career (reprinted from *Musing of the Great Blue* blog, Clark, 2012b).

My Mentor and Me: A True Story

More than 30 years ago, I started my first nursing position—it was a dream job for an energetic and eager, newly minted nurse. I worked on a surgical floor where my major responsibilities included educating and preparing patients for their surgical procedures and caring for them after they returned. I loved my job, my patients, my colleagues, and my free time! I began my shift at 5 a.m. and ended at 1 p.m. In good weather, I rode my bicycle, because I didn't own a car, and during the harsh winters of the upper Midwest, I rode to work in a taxi driven by a trusted cabbie. My hours were awesome—especially for a young, single person who loved to recreate and be outdoors. But, like so many times in life, change happens.

About a year and a half into my job, the hospital hired a new director of nursing. I have to believe that her heart was in the right place and that she was doing what she thought was best for the hospital and the patients, but for me, her decisions would be life-changing. She decided, for reasons that still perplex me, to reassign many of the nurses to various units according to seniority and date of hire. Though I was thoroughly enjoying and thriving in my role on the surgical unit, I was one of the nurses reassigned. I was moved to the evening shift on what was then known as the "terminal unit." It was a dismal setting compared to where I had been working, and because I was a morning person, to me this was a death sentence. But very quickly, I grew to love my teammates and our patients, and I was surprised to discover that I had a knack for being present and listening to patients' stories. Many patients were in the end stages of their illnesses and in various phases of the dying process. I was a highly competent nurse, but I clearly needed improvement in my timeliness and efficiency. I discovered, as did my charge nurse, that because I enjoyed engaging in prolonged conversations with my patients, my task completion was often lacking. My charge nurse genuinely liked me and believed I was a skilled nurse, but on many occasions, she was compelled to remind me to complete my work on time. I realized that I needed to improve my timeliness, and I was working on it; yet, some nights I still fell short of my goals. And then one night, I experienced a defining moment in my young career.

It was late in the shift. The night in question was a busy one, and one of my tasks was to remove the irrigation apparatus from an elderly male patient who had recently undergone surgery for a transurethral resection. This type of surgery required an elaborate series of bottles and tubing, including a urinary catheter inserted through the male genitalia and progressing into the bladder, where fluids could be used for irrigation. The charge nurse asked me to remove the apparatus and to do it with expediency, because we had much more work to be done. I was determined to show how well I could perform the skill and to do it in a swift and efficient manner. I walked into the patient's room, greeted him, and began to explain the procedure. He gazed at me with tired eyes and asked, "Will it hurt?"

I paused and then said gently, "Of course, I'm not a man, but when I have done this procedure for other gentlemen, they have told me it is pretty uncomfortable."

He responded, "I'm not ready yet—can we talk for a while?" So, I sat beside him and we talked. He had recently lost his wife of many decades.

He spoke of her that night—he talked about their life together, their children, and how aggrieved he was when his beloved wife took her final breath. We talked for about 10 minutes, and then he said he was ready. I briefly explained the procedure and went about removing the tubing and disengaging the apparatus. I started to say good night when I noticed tiny unshed tears in the corners of his eyes. I couldn't just leave, so I sat with him for a few more minutes. Then, I gathered the equipment, and as I was rolling it down the hall, I bolstered myself for a "talking to" by my charge nurse. Clearly, I had not performed my responsibilities in the desired time frame. Sure enough, as I walked down the hallway, I was met by my charge nurse, who politely asked me to dispose of the equipment, finish my assigned responsibilities, and to meet her in the conference room after completing our shift.

Believe me, I was pretty worried. I prepared myself for the possibility for that night to be my last. After our shift, we entered the conference room. The charge nurse gently closed the door, folded her hands, and said, "Cindy, you have missed your calling. I want you to think seriously about going back to school to become a psychiatric nurse. You have a genuine gift for being present with people and listening with real compassion and interest." And then she sat back quietly in her chair. Imagine my surprise. I looked at her, acknowledged her suggestion, and promised her that I would give it serious thought. I reflected on our conversation and realized she was right. I began making plans to return to school to become a psychiatric nurse. And she was right—I loved my clinical career as a psychiatric nurse for many years before becoming a nursing professor. I am forever grateful and will never forget the care shown to me by my charge nurse who saw something in me that I did not. Rather than reprimand or discourage me, or suggest that I find another position, she shined a light on a pathway of new discovery that launched a fabulous career in psychiatric nursing.

I learned many lessons from that experience. I learned that when we look for what's right and good, and when we genuinely care about someone, we can change people's lives. In the course of my own career, I have tried to model my charge nurse's guidance bestowed on me more than 35 years ago. I looked for and celebrated the strengths of my patients when I worked as a clinical nurse, and I try to do the same for my students in my faculty role. These valuable lessons have made and continue to make an impression on how I view and navigate the world.

Introducing Best Practices in Academic Mentoring

Nick et al. (2012) expanded the work of the National League for Nursing (2006b) to introduce six major themes of "mentoring" best practices aimed at establishing a formal academic mentoring program. The six themes are:

1. Achieving appropriately matched dyads

2. Establishing clear mentorship purpose and goals

3. Solidifying the dyad relationship

4. Advocating for and guiding the protégé (mentee)

5. Integrating the protégé into the academic culture

6. Mobilizing institutional resources

The authors attest that relationships play a key role in any successful mentorship experience and contend that mentoring programs contribute to improved faculty morale, higher career satisfaction, and increased self-confidence in professional development. Further, the authors conclude that mentored faculty publish more, obtain more grants, and are promoted more quickly. They also say that institutions that provide mentoring programs experience increased retention, an improved sense of community and professional identity, and faculty members who are better positioned to navigate the academic environment and can more easily transition to new roles and responsibilities. Ultimately, successful mentoring moves the profession forward and can have a positive impact on faculty career attainment, institutional culture, and leadership development.

Unfortunately, we face a scarcity of qualified and available mentors. Mentoring relationships are plagued by time constraints, unrealistic expectations, poor or incomplete preparation, and, sadly, competitiveness or a desire to "clone" oneself. The most effective mentoring relationships are built on trust and collaboration; career advancement or revitalization; and reciprocal respect, sharing, and caring. For most of us, our achievements can be attributed to the power of positive mentorship—the heroes who have encouraged us to hope, to never settle, to set goals, and to pursue our dreams. We are all "standing on the shoulders of giants," and by doing so, we see more and accomplish more, because they raise us up. My mentors have all been great teachers—giants, if you will—who each in their own personal and profound ways have been a blessing in my life. As the English author and dramatist George Colman noted, "Praise the bridge that carried you over."

Unfortunately, we also have cynics in our lives who seek to diminish us and mock our dreams of a desired future. We must make every effort to deflect their discouragement and reinterpret their pessimism to energize us, focus us, and inspire us to achieve our goals. This can best be accomplished by aligning ourselves with positive mentors and role models who encourage and inspire us. As one of my mentors said to me, "Why soar at 30,000 feet when you can soar at 60,000 feet?" We need to show gratitude to those who helped us soar at 60,000 feet and then "pay it forward" by modeling the way and mentoring others, and encouraging them to live a purposeful life.

Deflecting or reframing criticism can be difficult, but with practice (and by engaging positive mentors), we can improve our "criticism-deflecting" abilities. I have included a personal example in the "Deflecting Criticism" sidebar.

DEFLECTING CRITICISM

The situation: *Several years ago, I was very excited to share a secret desire to pursue a major (and, I might add, challenging and lofty) goal with another professor. I'll call her Professor Grim. Professor Grim had achieved the same goal several years earlier, so of course, I thought she was the very best person to advise me on how to proceed in my pursuit. She agreed to join me for lunch so we could strategize my course of action. As I laid out my plan, her nonverbal language spoke volumes. She fidgeted and failed to make eye contact. When I asked for her opinion about ways to reach my goal, she chuckled and said that it was a long shot. She explained that I was undeserving because I had not accomplished nearly enough during my nursing career and told me to forget about it. I was flabbergasted.*

I spent way too much time over the course of the next year or more thinking about our conversation. It took a long time for me to realize that she did not have my best interests in mind and for me to reframe her discouragement. Finally, I woke up and realized that I had consulted a naysayer (or tormentor) instead of a mentor. That same day, I contacted one of the most famous nurse leaders in the country, asking for her opinion of my pursuit of this goal. She was not only encouraging but also an incredible and inspiring coach. With her guidance and generous support, I succeeded in reaching this pivotal goal.

Reframing a situation can sometimes be difficult, especially if we have been targeted by an uncivil person or made to feel insignificant and unimportant or unworthy. At these times, we must take a deep breath, check in with people who genuinely have our best interest in mind, and help us reevaluate the merits of the messages we have received.

Other tips:

1. *First, consider the source—have you engaged a naysayer or a trusted mentor?*

2. *If you have engaged a naysayer, take a deep breath and say something like, "I appreciate your opinion and I will give it some thought." Upon reflection, if the person's opinion has merit, consider it; but if not, simply discard the comments and move on.*

3. *If it is clear that the naysayer is deliberately trying to offend or insult you, you might say, "It seems that you are intentionally trying to offend me. Because we are colleagues, I would appreciate being treated more respectfully—and you can expect the same from me."*

4. *If you are conferring with a trusted mentor or with a person who sincerely cares about you, try not to take personal offense to the person's feedback. Instead, look for the lesson and seek advice on specific steps you can take to position yourself for future success.*

Finishing Touches

Creating and living a powerful and compelling personal, professional vision; being an inspiring role model; and serving as an encouraging and motivating mentor gives our lives meaning and purpose. As we construct and solidify the principles that undergird our lives, we are building a life of significance and consequence. True leadership calls for living a principled and examined life, reflecting on our own vision and purpose of a desired future, and practicing daily habits of civility and respect. Engaging trusted mentors in this journey is critical to our personal and professional growth and developent. I appreciate the alluring words of author and poet Maya Angelou: "I've learned that people will forget what you said, people will forget what you did, but people will never forget how you made them feel."

CIVILITY TIP

Think about the characteristics you admire or look for in a trusted mentor. Do you want a skilled listener who is candid, caring, and nonjudgmental—someone who is able to give and receive constructive feedback, ask probing and compelling questions, and be generous with time and wisdom? If so, these may also be the traits you wish to develop in yourself as you "pay it forward" by mentoring others.

Chapter 7
Pathway for Fostering Organizational Civility: Institutionalizing Change

When you're finished changing, you're finished. –Benjamin Franklin

This chapter discusses:

- Raising awareness
- Assembling a civility team
- Planning a civility strategy
- Assessing the plan and celebrating success

Setting the Stage for Organizational Civility

All organizations, including nursing programs, possess a unique culture with distinctive beliefs, principles, and values. The culture of any organization is closely linked to employee satisfaction, recruitment, and retention, because the ways in which employees perceive their workplace often drives how they act and behave. Creating and sustaining a civil work environment improves communication, teamwork, individual and organizational trust, and job satisfaction. Several factors can affect the culture of any organization, including level of job satisfaction, employee commitment, and turnover rates—all directly related to the interaction between employees and their ability to do the job, their loyalty to the organization, and the level of support they experience from the leaders of the organization (Mathis & Jackson, 2008).

> **NOTE**
>
> *In the original version of this book, the Pathway for Fostering Organizational Civility (PFOC) was presented in Chapter 11. In this edition, I have chosen to introduce the PFOC earlier in the text because I fundamentally believe that real and meaningful change only occurs by purposefully and intentionally attending to (and potentially transforming) the culture and social architecture of the organization.*

Reengineering and redesigning the organizational culture requires that we be vigilant to factors that contribute to organizational demise—impaired communication, low morale, negative attitudes, and poor performance—then take bold action to initiate and sustain organizational change (Springer, Clark, Strohfus, & Belcheir, 2012). All of this takes hard work, focus, commitment, and strong, effective leadership at all levels of the organization. The desired result is a transformed organization that faculty, students, and administrators enjoy and celebrate. Incremental changes are generally inadequate to renovate the culture; instead, transformational change involves completely redesigning how the organization is structured and managed, redefining its vision and goals, and establishing new norms, systems, and practices (Bigelow & Arndt, 2005).

Though no universal, one-size-fits-all framework for fostering organizational civility and achieving a healthy workplace exists, several essential components can be implemented to increase the potential for doing so. Any model or pathway to foster civility must be considered within the context of the organization's unique culture and climate, and must be nimble and flexible enough to use in a variety of work environments.

Metaphor of the Aspen Grove

Margaret Wheatley (1994) reminds us that organizations have an organic and natural tendency to change and evolve. They self-organize, and as such, change is viewed as power, capacity, and unfolding movement toward new forms of order and patterns of creativity and growth. Organizations are adaptable and order-seeking and, if healthy, create diversity and connectedness. Each time we influence the system (organization), we are creating possibilities for change and transformation. The world is a co-created one, where no individual exists in isolation and where the workplace is a constant flow of interaction, communication, and relationships between and among individuals. We continuously affect one another as well as being affected by the organization in which we work. Organizations are living systems, and fostering positive change is an organic process that ultimately proliferates and thrives. Thus, the imagery and energy of an aspen grove provides a powerful metaphor for positive and sustained organizational change. Like an aspen grove, the process for fostering organizational civility might begin with a single seedling of change that then grows and spreads by sending out runners that take deep root to fortify and reinforce the strength of the system. When we look closely, we see that the aspen grove is one vast, incredible connection.

Extending the aspen metaphor with the Pathway for Fostering Organizational Civility (PFOC), the seedling or the impetus for change can take on many forms, ranging from an individual initiative, to dissatisfaction with the status quo, to a pre-established intention to improve the organizational culture. With commitment and support, the seedling for change can thrive and prosper, becoming a catalyst for further organizational change, emerging into a cyclical process in which new seedlings of change initiatives are created to enrich, reinvigorate, and sustain the system. Ultimately, civility becomes an integral part of the work environment and firmly embedded in the organizational culture.

To achieve transformational change, I have developed an evidence-based, eight-step process (PFOC) to help organizational leaders and teams create and sustain healthy, civil work environments. Figure 7.1 illustrates the PFOC.

Pathway for Fostering Organizational Civility [PFOC]

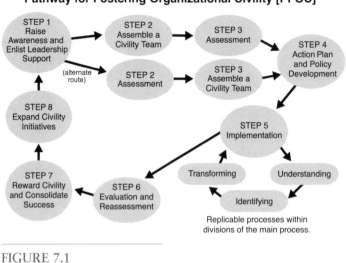

FIGURE 7.1

Pathway for Fostering Organizational Civility.

Creating Organizational Civility

Many academic institutions are faced with transforming the work environment from one of incivility to civility. The main goal of the Pathway for Fostering Organizational Civility (PFOC) is to help teams and organizations to create healthier and more civil workplaces. This comprehensive and dynamic approach to workplace improvement engages employees, leaders, and stakeholders at myriad levels and provides a fluid and progressive step-by-step process to promote collegiality, teamwork, and collaboration—and ultimately a culture of civility and respect.

Step 1: Raise Awareness and Enlist Leadership Support

Raising awareness about the types and frequency of incivility is a vital step in fostering a civil organizational culture. This awareness often comes from faculty, staff, and students whose experiences are closest to the identified issue or problem and who are dissatisfied with the current state of the organization. These individuals help leaders and other members of the organization understand and appreciate the costs of uncivil actions, and in most cases, possess a vision of a better academic and work environment and a desire for positive change. Because transformational and sustained change requires broad-based collaboration, individuals need support from leaders, administrators, and key stakeholders who share a similar vision and who have the necessary resources to support the change. Raising awareness about incivility and its harmful effects and expressing a sincere desire for change can be powerful motivators to transform the culture and enlist support from leaders.

Enlisting the support of leaders and administrators is essential not just because they have access to necessary resources, but also because they have a vested interest in the organization and frequently possess a broader view. Their knowledge of the workplace and experience with previous and current incivility issues can help substantiate potential problems and provide insight into possible solutions. Because leaders oversee the organization and have the capacity to allocate resources, their support is vital to successful organizational change. In addition, their experience with past attempts to address incivility, if any, can provide valuable lessons.

When meeting with leaders and administrators to enlist support, you need to keep certain key elements in mind. First, be prepared to share your own and others' experiences with incivility—the information must be objective, clearly documented, and substantiated. Obtain their perspective of workplace incivility issues and inquire about past or current initiatives to address the problem. If the leaders are aware of the incivility problem and have a current initiative in place to foster organizational civility, offer to be part of the change process. If the leaders are aware of the incivility problem but have no current initiative in place or if the leaders are unaware of the incivility problem, suggest implementing the PFOC and the installation of a Civility Team (aka an Organizational Culture Team, a Design Team, or any other suitable name determined by the team members with input from others) to measure and address the problem. Provide rationale for a civility initiative, determine the level of leadership support, and appraise and secure resources needed to effect cultural change. If an assessment of organizational culture and civility has already been obtained, the Civility Team can oversee the implementation of a comprehensive civility initiative.

The overall goal is to institute or revise a shared governance model; identify teams (including a Civility Team); allocate responsibility and legitimate decision-making authority to teams; determine areas of strength and concern (low assessment scores) to be addressed by the Civility Team and other governance teams; develop and implement a strategic plan with action steps; chart progress; update others by providing open forums to discuss progress; seek input; and determine which items on the action plan require a "full vote."

Steps 2 and 3 can be reversed depending on whether an organizational assessment has already been conducted. If one has not been done, a Civility Team needs to be developed and charged with moving the civility initiative forward. If several employees share the same concern for workplace incivility and possess a similar vision of creating a more civil work environment, they might become members of the Civility Team (Step 2) and participate in the organizational culture and civility assessment (Step 3). If no clearly identified team members are available, you could obtain a consultant, appoint members of a Civility Team or voluntarily assemble them, or a combination of both, and charge them with assessing the organizational culture and level of civility (Step 3, then Step 2). Results of the assessment(s) will provide objective information about the scope of the problem, the strengths of the organization, insight and direction for positive change, and encouragement for members of the organization to support the development of a healthier workplace.

Step 2: Assemble a Civility Team: Seek Broad-Based Support

The Civility Team is charged with leading the transition to a more civil, healthy organizational culture. The team usually consists of five to seven members who are trusted, committed, and empowered to measure the problem, determine the strengths of the organization, develop a compelling vision of the organization's future, and carry out the steps of the PFOC. As previously mentioned, Civility Team members might be volunteers, selected from a pool of formal and informal leaders, or a combination of both. Members should represent rich and diverse ideas, a commitment to the vision, and dedication to teamwork and collaboration. Members of the Civility Team should include an individual who holds a formal leadership position and individuals who are fully committed to the civility initiative. Certain members should be avoided—people with inflated egos, who generate mistrust and hinder teamwork, and who undermine and/or sabotage fulfilling the goals for change. I highly recommend that the Civility Team be given equal status as other teams/committees within the nursing program. Doing so provides a formal structure for team functioning including bylaws, policies and procedures for committee functioning, and reporting responsibilities.

OUR LIVED EXPERIENCE AS A CIVILITY TEAM

During my tenure as a faculty member, we assembled a Civility Team (aka Culture Team) in our school of nursing (SON). The team was composed of six diverse members—both genders, tenured and non-tenured faculty, classified staff, clinical faculty, and research faculty were all represented. Some of us were recruited by the director, others volunteered, and all of us were happy to serve. I was the team facilitator, though everyone played a critical and important role. We developed a team charter with team norms, and agreed that "the only skin we had in the game was to develop an excellent product and move the school forward." The team members were enthusiastic, smart, dedicated, and focused on quality. Our main charge was to identify areas for improvement and strength based on our scores of organizational assessment gathered over a 10-year period. We assessed five main areas of organizational culture: teamwork, communication, decision-making, conflict, and work satisfaction. We also measured three contextual areas: overall morale, personal level of stress, and perceived amount of change. In one of the assessments conducted in 2011, we noted some changes in our overall scores. Some of our scores dropped—not a lot, but we knew we needed to explore the matter further. The team conducted an organizational root cause analysis (RCA) using the 5 Whys Approach—a simple, effective tool to identify the root cause of a problem. Using this approach, we were able to isolate the problem, determine ways to address it, reinforce areas of strength, and engage faculty and staff in the ongoing initiative.

High-performing teams don't happen automatically or by happenstance. Too often, individuals are asked to serve on a team with little attention paid to competencies of high-performing teams. Think about it, how often have team members been selected based on convenience, availability, and because "it's your turn" or "there's no one to fill this position"? Team selection should be thoughtful, purposeful, and based on achieving the competencies of high-performing teams. To achieve high performance status, teams need time to form, storm, norm, and perform (Tuckman, 1965). This progressive development requires time, effective leadership, commitment to a shared purpose, a focus on relationships, accountability and trustworthiness, focus on quality and results, and well-honed communication and conflict-negotiation skills.

COMPETENCIES OF HIGH-PERFORMING TEAMS

1. *Share a common vision, purpose, direction*

2. *Establish and commit to a Team Charter with team norms*

3. *Foster interpersonal and organizational trust*

4. *Utilize effective problem-solving and decision-making skills*

5. *Invite feedback and varying opinions and perspectives*

6. *Be productive, with a dual focus on process and achieving results*

7. *Clarify roles for all team members*

8. *Utilize constructive communication and conflict negotiation*

Obtaining team commitment and supporting leadership development for the members of the Civility Team are key elements in Step 2. Because any sustained change requires prolonged and substantial effort, time, and energy, team members and leaders need to understand and appreciate the scope of the commitment Civility Team members are being asked to undertake. Incentives such as workload adjustments can be offered to encourage team involvement. Administrators must empower and assign the Civility Team the responsibility, legitimate authority, and decision-making power for carrying out the steps and initiatives included within the PFOC. Without this power and authority, the Civility Team lacks the ability and authorization to legitimately promote change. Members need to build and/or deepen their team commitment to move the initiative forward and link their personal, professional values and vision to those of the civility initiative, thus drawing energy from their individual and collective beliefs.

Objectives of the Civility Team include:

1. **Participate in leadership development initiatives to strengthen individual and team leadership potential and skill sets**

By virtue of their membership on the Civility Team, the members are leaders and, as such, are charged with communicating a vision of the desired culture, inspiring commitment, recognizing individual and collective contributions, delegating needed resources, and ensuring that plans are followed through to completion. However, many people who assume leadership positions lack sufficient leadership skills and experience to perform those tasks. As a result, an initiative to foster organizational civility and change should be coupled with leadership training. Team members must be given adequate time and resources to develop and practice leadership skills, such as assuming and delegating responsibilities, negotiating conflict, collaborating, conducting successful meetings, utilizing effective measurement tools, interpreting and summarizing assessment findings, communicating, and generating reports.

2. **Appraise individual and team commitment and availability of personal, collective, and organizational resources**

Determine how and when meetings will take place, set meeting times, determine team roles and responsibilities, and establish a timeline and cost structure of initiative development while still allowing a reasonable margin of error. The goal is to foster a healthy climate for teamwork—one that has a sense of community, shared vision, and positive outlook and one that encourages teammates to model their commitment for the desired change. One of the most important aspects of team cohesion is co-creating team norms.

3. **Co-create a team charter with team norms and build in accountability measures**

A team charter is a detailed document that is developed with input from all members of the team early during team formation and referred to (and revised as needed) over the life span of the team. Team charters clarify the team's purpose and direction and clearly delineate processes, responsibilities, and deliverables. The charter is agreed to, and it represents "buy-in" from the members. Team charters typically include the following elements:

- Team members/roster
- Team purpose and goals
- Roles and responsibilities
- Key objectives/deliverables
- Decision-making processes
- Team communication processes
- Ground rules/team norms

An essential aspect of the charter is the establishment of team norms. The norms are important parameters for effective team functioning and should stem from the organization's vision, mission, philosophy, and shared values. Without functional norms, desired behavior is ill-defined, and thus, team members are left to "make things up as they go along." To co-create norms, the Civility Team must dedicate sufficient time to ask all team members to brainstorm behaviors that lead to effective team functioning and contribute to a healthy work environment. Be sure to avoid critiquing the suggestions; let the ideas flow. Then brainstorm behaviors that *do not* lead to effective team functioning. After the desirable and undesirable behaviors have been identified and agreed upon, the team can develop and affirm norms. Some common examples of norms include how each team member will communicate, resolve conflicts, be accountable for fulfilling individual and collective responsibilities, and conduct themselves in meetings. As soon as the norms are agreed upon, they become the standard for team interactions, and they need to be reviewed, revisited, and revised on a regular basis.

The team needs to examine each individual's values and beliefs and co-create team norms that reflect the desired organizational and cultural change. Then, the members need to determine how norms can be operationalized and how each team member can "live" the norms. This requires individual and collective accountability. Holding yourself and others accountable is critical to every successful organization. Accountability (or lack thereof) is closely associated with defining goals, knowing what is expected to reach them, and agreeing to hold one another accountable for the desired results. I like Miller's SIMPLE solution (Miller, n.d.) for building and sustaining accountability—it goes like this:

S–Set Expectations: All members of the organization need to know what is expected of them before they can be held accountable. The organization must clearly state upfront the expectations and goals, including when, how, and to what level of quality the goals are to be accomplished.

I–Invite Commitment: After goals and expectations are set, each person needs to commit to achieving them. Buy-in is more likely if people understand how the goals and expectations benefit them personally, and how the goals will move the organization forward. This connection is imperative to accepting the goals and holding one another accountable for the results.

M–Measure Progress: Measures to determine whether or not employees are meeting the goals and expectations are critical to holding people accountable. Progress toward goal achievement (e.g., meeting the established norms) can be included in a 360° evaluation that includes feedback from team members, peers, administrators, and self-assessment data.

P–Provide Feedback: Setting clear expectations coupled with quality feedback is the backbone of holding someone accountable. Providing constructive feedback regarding areas of strength and improvement isn't foolproof; however, it opens the door for problem-solving and follow-up actions. In many cases, giving objective, sincere feedback with a desire to support the employee is sufficient to change behavior.

L–Link to Consequences: If employees are meeting the expectations and goals of the organization, praise and reward their achievements. If employees are not meeting the goals they committed to, determine if they have an ability problem (i.e., they do not have the skills to complete the task). In this case, they might require more training. If they face a motivation problem, coaching, redirection, or issuing a consequence might help them deliver on their commitment. Consequences must be fair and appropriate. This is not a punitive measure, but instead a measure to encourage employees to take commitments more seriously.

E–Evaluate Effectiveness: Review the goals and determine if they are useful in holding employees accountable for reaching those goals. Be sure to review how the process was handled and identify ways to be more effective at applying the principles of holding one another accountable.

4. Identify empirical measures, assessment strategies, and benchmarks for organizational civility and success (See Step 3)

5. Determine resources, timeline, and cost structure for the civility initiative while allowing a reasonable margin of error (See Step 3)

6. Enlist broad-based support for the civility initiative from leaders, faculty, staff, students, and community partners

Enlisting broad-based support means engaging people at all levels of the organization, communicating clearly and widely, and encouraging all members of the organization to participate and work together to achieve the desired vision. Information about the civility initiative and its progress can be communicated internally and externally via face-to-face meetings, web pages, memos, newsletters, and through formal meeting minutes. Eliminate "silos" that discourage communication, and reduce the existence of pet projects and sacred cows, so that "the way we've always done things" does not impede achieving the desired vision. This might include redesigning systems to support the desired change and providing incentives for civility. With broad-based support and buy-in, the civility initiative is more likely to succeed.

Step 3: Assess Organizational Culture and Civility at All Levels

Because every organization possesses a unique history, culture, and workforce, careful and thorough assessment can provide meaningful information to individualize the civility initiative, thus increasing the chance of success. First, the Civility Team should select an evidence-based, valid, and reliable tool to conduct pre- and post-test assessments of organizational culture and civility. The post-test assessment will be conducted on an ongoing interval basis to measure and evaluate the progress of the civility initiative. Some examples of measurement tools include:

- Healthy Work Environment Inventory (Clark, Sattler, & Barbosa-Leiker, 2016)

- Organizational Civility Scale (OCS) (Clark, Landrum, & Nguyen, 2013)

- Culture/Climate Assessment Scale (CCAS) (Clark, Belcheir, Strohfus, & Springer, 2012)
- Civility/Incivility-specific instruments:
  - Incivility in Nursing Education-R [INE-R] (Clark, Barbosa-Leiker, Gill, & Nguyen, 2015)
  - Workplace Incivility/Civility Survey [WICS] (FKA Faculty-to-Faculty Incivility Survey) (Clark, 2013; Clark, Olender, Kenski, & Cardoni, 2013)
  - Incivility in Online Learning Environment [IOLE] (Clark, Ahten, & Werth, 2012; Clark, Werth, & Ahten, 2012)
- Civility, Respect, Engagement in the Workforce (CREW) Scale (Osatuke, Moore, Ward, Dyrenforth, & Belton, 2009)

After a measurement tool has been selected, the team should conduct an in-depth analysis of the factors that influence organizational culture and civility. Personnel at all levels of the organization should participate in the pre- and post-test assessments. In addition to the assessment data, the Civility Team can use formal and informal reports, notes, evaluations, records (of past failed/successful attempts), satisfaction surveys, regulatory reports, Equal Employment Opportunity (EEO) records (if discoverable), interviews, focus groups, and open forums to augment the assessment information. Maintaining and ensuring confidentiality and integrity of the assessment data and upholding all human subject protocols are critical. Likewise, the team can also use external researchers and firms to collect, analyze, and report the assessment findings, thus establishing a study less likely to be biased. The Civility Team is also charged with completing a three-pronged analysis of the organization including a focused analysis, programmatic analysis, and a cultural analysis.

Focused Analysis

After a careful and comprehensive review of the assessment data, the Civility Team will generate focused analyses and a summary of the findings. These focused analyses might encompass the human and economic costs of uncivil behaviors, the greatest human benefits and economic returns from successful change, parameters by which the economic and human impact can be measured, and benchmarks by which behaviors/behavioral change can be measured.

Programmatic Analysis

Programmatic analysis examines how change efforts should be organized and managed to maximize the likelihood of success. This process focuses on the group dynamics and the pace by which the group and the organization as a whole react to change. Some groups respond better to rapid change, whereas others require a more structured and steady approach. Likewise, in some organizations, formal leaders are well-positioned to guide the change, whereas other organizations might be successfully led through a grassroots approach. The Civility Team can obtain important information from records of past attempts and from comparable change initiatives from similar organizations. Ultimately, the Civility Team will assess individual and organizational responses to previous changes; identify the key individuals who need to be involved in the change process; select effective leaders to manage and oversee the process; determine the structure, composition, and purposes of committees and/or teams; identify the best theoretical model(s) and strategies to introduce and mobilize the change process; and determine an appropriate and functional timeline for the overall civility initiative.

Cultural Analysis

This analysis involves the study of various cultural factors that influence individual and collective perceptions and reactions to the environment and to the proposed changes. These factors most often impact individuals on a subconscious level and include the following:

1. **Values:** Deeply held beliefs about the appropriate way to behave—personal principles and standards that individuals construct for themselves.

2. **Norms:** Expected and accepted behavior in the workplace. These are the group standards and codes of conduct that individuals co-create and accept.

3. **Organizational support systems:** Laws, rules, policies, procedures, guidelines, and the "grapevine." These are the formal and informal tenets that govern the workplace.

4. **Peer support:** Encouragement and collaboration from coworkers who celebrate successes and provide emotional/mental/psychological support, relationship-building, mentoring, role-modeling, and a sense of teamwork.

5. **Climate:** The invisible network or fabric that holds the workplace together. It includes working conditions, supervision, and interpersonal relationships. Climate can be studied in terms of:

   a. **A sense of community:** A sense of belonging and an awareness that others matter and add value to the organization, and that the individual, in turn, has a responsibility to be thoughtful to others

   b. **A shared vision:** Recognition that members of the organization possess similar values and goals, which leads to a sense of inclusion, and that all members of the organization matter

   c. **A positive outlook:** Empowering people to seek opportunities rather than obstacles, and to search for strengths rather than deficits in one another and in the organization

Findings from the assessments and analyses can be used to individualize the civility initiative, including development and implementation of strategies, policies, and activities.

Step 4: Develop Plans, Policies, and Strategies

In this step, the Civility Team consolidates the information obtained from Step 3 and translates it into meaningful strategies, action plans, and policies that will be implemented in Step 5. Consolidating the assessment data and summarizing the findings can be used to generate an overarching and compelling vision for the civility initiative and organizational change. To do this, the team might find the following actions helpful:

1. **Consider the organization's vision**—Is it shared? Does the vision inspire action? Does the vision need to be revised? Can individuals articulate the vision? Do they share a sense of community and collegiality, and do they believe that organizational change is possible? Do individuals share a vision for civility and respect? Have they bought into the desired vision, and are they committed to the civility initiative? If not, does a new vision need to be created or the current vision revised? If so, various frameworks for creating an organizational vision exist; Latham's (1995) is my favorite because it provides a clear, systematic structure for creating a collective and shared vision of

the future. Please see Chapter 5 for details and a step-by-step process for creating an organizational vision. After agreement is reached on a desired vision of civility, the team must share it broadly and widely with all members and stakeholders of the organization.

2. **Review the data and assessment findings and consider them within the context of the organization**—Emphasis is placed on improving organizational civility; however, individual effort and commitment are also needed to achieve sustained results.

3. **Identify areas of strength and excellence**—Reinforce and celebrate efforts already in place to enhance a civil workplace.

4. **Determine and implement specific strategies to improve areas of concern and to reinforce areas of strength**—Each strategy should include clear objectives, expected timelines, the necessary resources (financial, human, and organizational) to implement and evaluate the strategies, individuals, or teams assigned to accomplish each strategy and desired results.

Policy development and implementation is critical to organizational change and to the success of the civility initiative. I developed the SMART policy as a framework to report and address incivility, to reward civility, and to evaluate progress.

The SMART policy applies to all circumstances where an act of incivility or bullying occurs among or between faculty, students, staff, administrators, community partners, or other relevant parties. The policy also provides a mechanism for documenting and rewarding civility. The steps are:

System for confidential reporting

Managing report information

Addressing incivility

Rewarding civility

Tracking and evaluating progress

System for Confidential Reporting

If a confidential reporting system does not exist within your institution, the Civility Team or designee can create one (Healthy Work Environment or Civility Policy) by which members and visitors of the workplace can report incidents of incivility (and civility). Anonymity of the reporters and validity and confidentiality of each report will be ensured. The report can be either a paper or an electronic document and can be accessible online from outside the institution. An employee or student ID, name, and contact information will be collected for statistical and follow-up purposes only and will not be released to any parties. Specific fields include time, date, and location of occurrence; description of the incident; impact of incivility; the reporter's perception of and response to the issues; and suggestions for follow-up. These data are valuable in determining the success of the PFOC by tracking incidents of civility and incivility and, if indicated, in imposing sanctions and/or follow-up actions for the offender.

Go to the following URL to see a sample reporting system: https://boisestate.qualtrics.com/SE/?SID=SV_82mxbb1Mjv95t52

Managing Report Information

Although the Civility Team (or designee) may be instrumental in assisting in the design and implementation of a confidential reporting system, it is not recommended that members of the Civility Team respond to the reports and/or issue sanctions if indicated. Other entities such as Human Resources personnel are better suited to examine the validity of the report by interviewing the individuals involved and providing follow-up procedures if needed. This ensures confidentiality for all parties involved.

Addressing Incivility

To the individual who bears witness to or is affected by uncivil behaviors: The emphasis is on using assertive, behavioral terms to address uncivil situations/disruptive behaviors. Subsequent to filing the incivility report, the individuals involved will meet with a supervisor or mediator to address and resolve the problem. Each person will alternate detailing his or her view of the situation, and each will adhere to stating objective information and speaking directly and respectfully to one another using "I" statements instead of "you" statements. The goal is to find an interest-based resolution, with clear expectations, and an agreement on who is going to do what by when. If individuals seek common ground and pursue a compromise, they are more likely to arrive at a win-win solution. A plan for a follow-up meeting to evaluate progress on efforts to resolve the issue will be established.

To the individual displaying uncivil behaviors: The emphasis for corrective actions will be placed on the behavior and not the person. The first violation of the policy will result in the employee getting a verbal warning and no written documentation placed in his or her employee file. Upon the second incivility infraction, the supervisor will initiate a Performance Improvement Plan (PIP). The PIP includes education regarding the financial, human, and organizational costs that result from disruptive behaviors; it also prescribes specific behavioral requirements (self-control classes, stress management, etc.) and associated time frames. If the person makes minimal or no improvement, or repetitive incidents are reported against that person, disciplinary actions such as suspension, temporary leave, etc., might be warranted. If the disruptive behavior is the result of a team or an organizational conflict, the supervisor will address the underlying issue(s) and make recommendations for resolution.

Rewarding Civility

The Civility Team (or designee) will create an evidence-based, confidential reporting system to collect reports of civility and acts of kindness and regard in the workplace. Reporters can identify themselves or remain anonymous. The report can be a paper or an electronic document and can be accessible online from outside the institution. An employee or student ID, name, and contact information will be collected so that rewards can be rendered. Specific fields include time, date, description of the civil or respectful act, the reporter's perception of and response to the issues, and suggestions for follow-up. These data are valuable in determining the success of the PFOC by enhancing workplace members' knowledge of civility and will be used to dispense a "civility" reward (from a "wish list" of rewards and incentives) that the individual desires and holds in high regard.

Tracking and Evaluating Progress

The Civility Team (or designee) will institute a method to evaluate the SMART policy, monitor progress, and use evaluation data to modify or improve processes to reach the desired results. Using de-identified information, the team needs to keep a record of every action or strategy to evaluate processes and to generate a formal report(s) to communicate progress on the SMART policy. The reports will be disseminated in aggregate to all members of the organization and used to keep leaders well-informed and to garner ongoing support for "staying on course" with the civility initiative.

Step 5: Implement Plans, Policies, and Strategies

The ultimate goal of the civility initiative is to foster organizational civility, to create civility champions to transform the workplace, to achieve sustainable results, and to garner support for continued change. Recall the metaphor of the aspen grove—though a single tree might be vulnerable to the forces of nature, a sturdy stand of aspen trees can withstand many hardships. Like the aspen grove, individuals within organizations must become part of a formidable, highly connected system of strength and transformation. Hence, the Civility Team will implement (or engage a Civility Expert to offer) a series of workshops with the goal of enabling participants to:

- Understand the undesired consequences of incivility and to realize the desired outcomes of a healthy, civil work environment

- Discuss an overview and summary of the organizational assessment data and findings

- Develop and implement evidence-based strategies to advance the civility initiative

- Secure a broad-based commitment to achieve and sustain a higher level of organizational civility and workplace health

The workshops will focus on three important subject areas—understanding, identifying, and transforming.

1. **Workshop—Understanding Focus:** Objectives include participants becoming familiar with the consequences of incivility on the existing organizational culture; the myriad human and economic costs of uncivil behaviors; and the essential elements of a healthy, civil workplace. Costs are presented in terms of their impact on individuals and teams as well as the organization, community, and society. The goal is for participants to

realize the impact of incivility and the goals of a civil work-place through visual, aural, and interactive experiences.

2. **Workshop—Identifying Focus:** Objectives include using em-pirical evidence to describe the impact of incivility by provid-ing an overview and a summary of the assessment data and findings. Participants are educated (or information is rein-forced) about the benefits of a civil organizational culture and workplace, the importance of developing a compelling and in-spirational vision, establishing and abiding by cultural norms, and identifying ways to ensure individual and organizational accountability. This information puts the focus on improving systems and reduces the likelihood of finger-pointing and in-dividual blame-placing. The workshop will reinforce the value of teamwork and collaboration to bring about meaningful results. Participants will also develop an understanding of and appreciation for the building blocks of culture: a shared vision, mission, philosophy, values, norms, organizational support systems, teamwork, and a solid strategic plan. Participants will be encouraged to share their experiences with incivility. Workshop facilitator(s) will provide clear parameters for shar-ing, discussing the impact of incivility, and involving the group in solution-focused approaches to recognize, address, and minimize incivility. Facilitator(s) will share and disseminate a clear and compelling organizational vision statement reflecting civility and respect by creating a picture or image of a desired culture: the type of workplace environment that supports and facilitates civility, promotes health, and achieves desired results.

3. **Workshop—Transforming Focus:** Objectives include partici-pants creating and agreeing to meaningful and achievable goals. The goal-setting activity should be done at both indi-vidual and organizational levels. The Clark Workplace Civility Index can be used to develop short- and long-term individual goals and objectives. Participants will work together to draft an organizational action plan. To facilitate the planning pro-cess, participants will be made aware of what is being done to date to bring about sustained change. New ideas will be gener-ated, and an action plan with measurable goals will be drafted by the participants. Specific outcomes include:

   - Develop and obtain buy-in for a positive and affirming statement of shared values. Consider what the organization values and does not value. Craft an organizing platform from which individual and collective actions are based.

- Introduce the **SMART** policy (described previously).
- Co-create norms of behavior based on vision and statement of shared values:
  - Participants will develop and adopt an action plan with measurable goals to cultivate and sustain civility. (See sidebar for an Action Plan template.) Civility and norm compliance is incorporated into the performance evaluation process (consider instituting a 360° feedback system) to build in accountability.
  - Participants will be made aware of what is being done to create and sustain change (for example, follow-up activities and an organizational support system to address/report incivility swiftly, directly, and fairly with consequences and sanction for violations).
  - At the same time, the Civility Team will reinforce and institute measures for personal and organizational civility.

ACTION PLAN TEMPLATE (EXEMPLAR)

Objective/Goal (To be accomplished)	Action (How objective/ goal will be met)	Responsible Party (Who is assigned to implement)	Time Frame for Completion or Implementation	Progress (Review regularly and sign-off when completed)

The workshops outlined in Step 5 can be repeated until your organization achieves the desired results. Use experiential and interactive strategies such as role-playing, simulations, and case studies to reinforce learning, teamwork, and accountability. A list of strategies for faculty, students, leaders, and organizations is provided in the sidebar that follows.

SUGGESTED STRATEGIES FOR FOSTERING ORGANIZATIONAL CIVILITY (LISTED IN NO PARTICULAR ORDER)

FACULTY-, LEADER-, AND STUDENT-FOCUSED APPROACHES

Acknowledge others and praise their work/contributions.

Acquire and work with a mentor(s) and coaches.

Apologize and mean it when the situation calls for it.

Assume goodwill, and expect the best from others.

Assume personal responsibility; hold yourself and one another accountable.

Attend meetings, arrive on time, participate, volunteer, and do your share.

Avoid abusing your position or authority.

Avoid distracting others (misusing media, side conversations) during meetings.

Avoid gossiping and spreading rumors.

Avoid making assumptions; clarify—ask questions and seek explanation and resolution.

Avoid taking credit for another individual's or team's contributions.

Bring your "A" game and a strong work ethic to the department, classroom, and clinical setting.

Co-create and abide by behavioral norms (department, team, classroom, clinical setting, etc.).

Communicate respectfully (by email, telephone, face-to-face) and really listen.

Conduct and participate in solution-focused open forums and governance teams.

Consider individual and team contributions to civil and uncivil interactions.

Demonstrate approachability, flexibility, and openness to other points of view.

Encourage, support, and mentor others.

Establish a professional vision and life plan; set personal and professional goals.

Exercise assertiveness; manage time wisely.

Include and welcome new and current colleagues/classmates.

Keep confidences and respect others' privacy.

Model civility, respectful social discourse, inclusion, and professionalism.

Participate in policy development, dissemination, and enforcement.

Participate on teams and committees.

Practice reflection exercises and keep a gratitude journal.

Practice self-care and stress-management techniques.

Practice, role-play, and simulate effective communication, constructive conflict negotiation, addressing incivility, teamwork and collaboration.

Role-model professionalism, inclusion, and respect.

Seek and encourage constructive feedback from others.

Share pertinent or important information with others.

Speak directly to the person with whom you have an issue.

Uphold the vision, mission, and values of the organization.

Use respectful language (avoid racial, ethnic, sexual, gender, and religiously biased terms).

continues

continued

ADDITIONAL FACULTY-FOCUSED APPROACHES
Attend civility workshops and increase teaching, classroom-management, and civility acumen.
Avoid showing favoritism.
Incorporate active and engaged teaching-learning strategies.
Incorporate behavioral objectives into courses.
Integrate civility into orientation, the nursing program, and curriculum.
Keep pace with and integrate technology into the teaching-learning environment.
Maintain confidentiality.
Publish teaching philosophies, clarify assignments, and reward good work.

ADDITIONAL STUDENT-FOCUSED APPROACHES
Attend class, be on time, and be prepared.
Avoid side conversations and monopolizing class.
Avoid distracting behaviors (for example, sleeping, checking email, surfing social networking sites, or working on assignments for another class).

LEADERSHIP- AND ORGANIZATIONAL-FOCUSED APPROACHES
Articulate a vision of civility and respect.
Avoid showing favoritism.
Celebrate and showcase faculty, staff, and student achievements.
Measure organizational culture, climate, and civility on an ongoing basis.
Implement an organizational civility initiative to improve workplace health.

Institute comprehensive civility training and education for all faculty, staff, and students.

Implement comprehensive, confidential reporting systems and policies.

Develop civility statements with shared values.

Hire (inspire) for civility (robust vetting of applicants).

Hire an ombud and/or civility liaison trained in civility.

Institute 360° evaluations.

Invest in post-exit interviews to discern "real" reasons for departure.

Maintain confidentiality.

Practice transparency.

Provide formal programming, training, and faculty/staff development:

    Cognitive rehearsal

    Constructive conflict negotiation

    Experiential activities and role-play

    Interactive videos and web-based programs

    Leadership development (emphasize management training)

    Listening, communicating, giving and receiving feedback

    Stress management

Provide mentoring and coaching programs.

Provide Web-based resources (guidelines, forms, references, experts).

Publicly convey decisions and rationale.

Reward civility.

Take complaints seriously and avoid making excuses for bad behavior.

Use empirical measurements for civility/incivility.

Step 6: Evaluation and Reassessment

Do not confuse activity with achievement. –Geno Auriemma, coach of the U.S. women's national basketball team

Simply because the Civility Team, leaders, and members of the organization have been active in their civility efforts does not mean that they have been successful. So you can be sure, you must measure and assess the elements of the PFOC. The PFOC is a cyclical process of assessing, planning, educating, strategizing, evaluating, and reassessing. As part of the cycle, evaluation and reassessment do not complete the pathway, but it is necessary to review the effectiveness of the change process to foster organizational civility. The Civility Team (or consultant) will re-administer the empirical and anecdotal measures to determine progress and goal achievement. Similarly, they will conduct focus groups and community forums to garner feedback from employees and other participants in the civility initiative. After the post-test data are gathered and summarized, the Civility Team will review the information and make recommendations for continuing the current measures and/or implementing revised actions and procedures to improve the organizational culture and level of civility.

Step 7: Reward Civility and Consolidate Successes

If you want something to grow, pour champagne on it! –Torben Rick

Though the PFOC is an ongoing process, you need to recognize and celebrate individual and collective achievements and successes all along the way. Doing so fuels momentum for change and rewards significant individual, team, and organizational efforts. This is related to the rewarding civility described in Step 4. The Civility Team will summarize and consolidate gains and embed civility into the organizational culture, as evidenced by:

- Shared and "lived" vision, mission, values, and norms

- Achievement of long- and short-term goals

- High morale, job satisfaction, and *esprit de corps*

- Strong recruitment and retention of faculty, staff, and students

- Skilled communication, collaboration, and decision-making

- Effective and reliable leadership

- Meaningful recognition of members

- Growth of new programs, initiatives, endowments, and revenue

- Career advancement

- Enhanced scholarly activity

- Increased visibility and community credibility

Step 8: Expand the Civility Initiative: Sharing Knowledge, Lessons, and Experience

After the evaluation process, the Civility Team (or designated facilitators) will conduct a transitional workshop for promising leaders and other interested parties to facilitate the passage of knowledge, lessons, and experience gained during the change process and implementation of the civility initiative. This phase includes 1) identifying leaders/members from the current Civility Team and 2) recruiting other interested team members to initiate the next phase of organizational civility.

1. **Leadership and team commitment:** In this phase, organizational leaders and members of the Civility Team will select new members—promising new leaders who are committed to ensuring cultural transformation, as well as those who openly express an interest in leading organizational change and becoming members of the expanded Civility Team. Their main charge will be to initiate and maintain the cultural change of fostering civility in the workplace.

2. **Sharing knowledge, lessons, and experience:** After selecting a team of new leaders, the Civility Team will organize a transitional workshop or retreat to provide new team leaders with an expanded view of the change process and how it can be improved and evaluated in future cycles. This process is integral to the recordkeeping discussed in Step 4. This is essentially a recap of the evaluation process, with the addition of future considerations:

   - What have we accomplished individually, collectively, and organizationally?

- What went well with the process? How can we continue and/or improve it?

- What didn't go well with the process? How can we correct it?

- Is the current situation aligned with the shared vision?

- If not, how can we apply the knowledge gained to meet the vision for civility?

At this point, the Civility Team has created and expanded a second-generation Civility Team that contributes to the continuation and development of the PFOC.

Hiring and Interviewing for Civility

Transforming the work environment, achieving and sustaining organizational excellence, emphasizing civility and respect, and creating positive workplaces are formidable attractors to recruit and retain the best and the brightest employees. Most, if not all of us, aspire to be part of a vibrant, healthy work environment where we are viewed as partners, valued as assets, and generously rewarded for our individual and collective contributions to the success of the organization (Clark, Sattler, and Barbosa-Leiker, 2016; Cipriano, 2011). We want to be affiliated with an organization on the rise, one that encourages free expression of diverse ideas, so that all voices might be heard and appreciated. We want to engage in work we enjoy, to reach our full potential, and to be part of a high-performing team.

Similarly, an important goal for all organizations it to avoid bringing incivility into the workplace in the first place and to stress civility and collegiality during the interview process. Group interviews can be especially helpful when interviewing applicants so that more than multiple perspectives are considered when onboarding potential colleagues. Whether you are a potential employer or employee, it is vital to ask relevant and important questions about the workplace culture during the interview process. I have provided a sampling of questions for both interviewees and interviewers.

Questions for interviewees to ask potential employers:

1. How does your organization live out its organizational vision, mission, and values? Give specific examples.

2. How would you describe the level of trust and quality of communication between leaders and other members of the organization? How does the leader's leadership style influence the workplace culture?

3. What policies has your organization established to address incivility and a negative work environment? How does the organization reward civility and professionalism?

4. Tell me about the organization's strategic approach to developing and sustaining a positive work culture.

5. Would you recommend this organization to your best friend or a family member as a good place to work?

6. If this organization could be summed up in one or two words, what would they be?

7. All things considered, is this a great place to work?

Questions for interviewers to ask of potential employees:

1. If we asked your former coworkers (students, supervisors) to describe your strengths/areas for improvement regarding collaboration and teamwork, what would they say? Give examples.

2. In what areas do you have the least amount of patience with coworkers (students, supervisors)? How do you express your impatience? Give examples.

3. What are your most significant contributions to promoting teamwork and collegiality among coworkers?

4. Describe a challenging situation or conflict you've experienced with a coworker (student, supervisor). What did you do about it? What was the outcome?

5. How do you see yourself contributing to the mission and values of the organization?

6. What feedback have you received about the style and impact of your interactions with coworkers (students, supervisors)? What insight have you gained from this feedback? What changes in your behaviors (if any) have you made as a result of this feedback?

7. Describe a high pressure situation you had to handle at work. What happened, who was involved, and what did you do to address the situation?

If you believe, as I do, that a positive work culture matters, then it is essential to take a proactive approach and be ready to ask some key questions that will help you make well-informed, responsible decisions regardless of which side of the interview process you reside on.

Finishing Touches

For the seeds of change to grow, spread, and transform into a fortified aspen grove, the pathway should continuously incorporate new data and information and evolve to a new pathway, much like how aspen trees absorb nutrients from the ground, the sky, and the air to expand and grow. This expansion and evolution can occur only when Civility Teams across the country and the globe come together and share their experiences. Because each organization's experience is unique and diversified, it might prove valuable for the community of civility leaders to collaborate on ongoing civility initiatives.

CIVILITY TIP

Hire for civility by asking applicants specific questions during the interview process. For example, you might ask, "In what areas do you have the least amount of patience in working with colleagues? How do you deal with your impatience?" Or you might ask, "If we asked your colleagues and students to describe your aptitude in the areas of collaboration, collegiality, and civility, what would they say?" A robust vetting of candidates can be a great start in building high-performance work teams and fostering a culture of civility.

Chapter 8
Fostering Effective and Meaningful Communication

I believe we can change the world if we start listening to one another. Simple, honest, human conversation…a chance to speak, to feel heard, and where we each listen well. It is the simple art of conversation that may ultimately save the world. –Margaret Wheatley

This chapter discusses:

- Defining and promoting effective communication
- Handling critical conversations in a civil way
- Engaging in conversations with students
- Addressing disruptive student behavior

Fostering Communication

We live in a high-tech, computerized (often stressful) information age where we are besieged with texts, emails, instant messages, phone calls, social media, and other technological communications that frequently leave us exhausted and overwhelmed. We send, receive, exchange, and process a vast amount of information every day. As faculty, especially if we teach online, our days are filled with exchanging information and making our best effort to communicate promptly and effectively with our students and colleagues. However, effective communication requires skill sets that go well beyond simply exchanging information. It involves a combination of verbal and nonverbal communication, active listening, and an awareness of our interactions with others. Interestingly, many individuals report greater difficulty engaging in face-to-face conversations than they have with electronic communication. Because nursing is a high-touch profession, nurses need to effectively communicate, and we must model this skill for our students. Effective communication can enhance relationships, improve teamwork, and possibly save our profession.

Engaging in meaningful and genuine conversation is one of the most potent tools in our toolbox for fostering civility. In Chapter 4, I detailed a study that I conducted to measure faculty perceptions of faculty-to-faculty incivility in nursing education. The findings from this study were compelling as well as perplexing. In one of the open-ended questions, I asked faculty to describe the most effective way to address and to deal with faculty-to-faculty incivility. After reading the first wave of stories, it became abundantly clear that faculty members were ill-prepared to deal with and effectively address incivility, especially with their peers and supervisors. Overwhelmingly, the respondents reported that using direct communication was the most effective strategy for addressing faculty-to-faculty incivility, yet most respondents commented on their reluctance to address issues head-on because they feared retaliation or felt ill-equipped to deal with incivility. Many requested faculty development workshops to learn to communicate effectively and to acquire the necessary skills to deal with the problem. Some respondents suggested that faculty development workshops, education, and use of civility consultants might help them learn ways to engage in direct, meaningful communication to effectively and constructively negotiate conflicted situations.

Conflicted situations and differences of viewpoint are inevitable, natural, normal processes which, when managed well, can lead to creative problem-solving. This is particularly true when problem-solving occurs in an atmosphere of civility, collaboration, and commitment to achieving a common purpose. Successfully negotiating conflict requires listening well and setting ground rules that provide a platform for acceptable conversation and interaction. In my work as a consultant, mastering the skills of conflict negotiation often tops the list of skill-building requests. Although many of us recognize that conflict can be a positive experience when it is addressed directly, we often avoid it, especially if a situation has evolved over time, bad feelings have built up, and relationships have been damaged—and in some cases, destroyed. In some instances, individuals avoid dealing with conflict because they lack the requisite skills or are unable to create the emotional "safe space" needed for effective dialogue and conflict resolution.

Other reasons for avoiding conflict include believing that mentioning the conflict or attempting to resolve it may put one's position or job at risk. Obviously, not all conflicts are created equal. Some may be resolved with a brief conversation that clears up misunderstandings, but others require work, energy, and willingness to revisit a painful issue. It is important, therefore, to decide which conflicts to address and which ones to let go.

Effective conflict negotiation requires that you carefully analyze your level of interest in the other party and how important it is to you to resolve the conflict. For example, if the issue is not of high interest to you or you are not deeply invested in the other party, the effort required to resolve the conflict may not be worth it. However, if the issue is of high interest to you and you are also highly invested in your relationship with the other party, it is probably in your best interest to attempt to resolve the problem, especially if both parties care about the results. It's important to realize that some problems or issues may never be resolved.

Though no universal techniques exist to successfully address incivility for every person in every situation, we can consider a few effective strategies. Engagement in critical conversations is one solution, but it must be done thoughtfully while making every attempt to avoid hastily or poorly expressed messages, impulsive responses, or misperceptions of intent. Each of us must consider the situation carefully before engaging in a critical communication. The following framework can help you prepare for and engage in a potentially thorny conversation in a civil way.

Reflecting, Probing, and Committing

To begin, assume that two faculty members are having a passionate disagreement over specific content to include or exclude in a nursing course they are teaching together. Each party vehemently disagrees on which subject matter to include, working together is becoming very stressful, and the faculty members are avoiding one another. Students are beginning to experience the consequences of this lack of cooperation, and they, too, are becoming confused and frustrated. I use this example to discuss dealing with these sorts of situations. When faced with the prospect of engaging in a potentially difficult conversation with a colleague, you need to ask yourself certain probing questions:

1. First, consider, "How important is my relationship with the other person?"

2. "If we are able to resolve the conflict, how much will it affect our working relationship now and in the future?"

3. After careful reflection, ask yourself, "If I don't address the conflict, will it negatively affect my ability to work with this person now and in the future?"

4. "How likely is it that the conflict will be resolved and the relationship improved?"

5. Lastly, ask, "What are the potential costs and benefits of addressing the situation?"

Once you have carefully considered these questions and have decided to address the conflict, you need to reflect and consider how you may have contributed to the situation. Even if you believe you had nothing to do with the conflict and the other person is to blame for the problem, in almost every case, this is not a true assessment. Even when it might be true, it's still important to consider the other person's point of view regarding your role. Doing so will help you develop an understanding of that person's perspective.

After you have pondered these questions and reflected on your role in the conflict, if you choose to engage in a conversation with your colleague, be sure to plan wisely. Creating emotional and physical safety and selecting the proper setting for this type of conversation should not be disregarded or underestimated. It should take place in a private area away from other people—assuming that no perceived threat to personal safety exists by having the conversation. If a threat to physical safety is perceived, enlist help from a trained mediator or a professional negotiator.

> **NOTE**
>
> *Consider meeting in a quiet place away from the noisy and fast-paced work environment. Select a place without interruptions and distractions. I enjoy conversations that take place outdoors—finding a walking path or a quiet park bench to chat can be very soothing and create a relaxing context for challenging conversations.*

Creating a Safe Zone

After you have reflected, probed, and made a decision to move forward, create a safe zone to conduct the conversation. First, attend to logistics. Both parties need to agree on a mutually beneficial time to meet in a quiet place without interruption. Before engaging in a potentially difficult conversation, allow the other party as much control as possible in making the arrangements. For example, email or call the other person asking whether and when he or she might be available for a conversation. You might say, "Jane, I realize that we have differences about our course content, and this disagreement has begun to affect our relationship, as well as our students. I am confident if we sit down and discuss some possible solutions, we can work this out together; please provide some possible dates and times and a place for us to meet. Thanks." Having the other party set the time and place for when and where the meeting will occur—hopefully away from the office and the busyness of the workplace—can diminish defensiveness and allows the other party to assert as much control as possible. (However, if you choose to have the other person select the meeting place, be sure to suggest a safe, quiet, relaxed venue conducive to conversation and problem-solving.) If desired, a third person can be invited by either side to listen in or mediate. After the meeting is set, think about how you might have contributed to the problem. This inventory will help you develop an understanding about the other person's perspective. The clearer we are about our goals and our role in the situation, the less we are controlled by fear and the more empowered we are to act.

At the outset of the meeting, setting ground rules (norms) and discussing common goals and interests are key. Establishing, agreeing upon, and abiding by behavioral norms and focusing on mutual interests help create a safe zone. Common norms include:

- Speaking one at a time
- Addressing the person directly
- Using a calm voice
- Avoiding personal attacks
- Using respectful language
- Sticking to objective information

Then, each party needs to agree on specific goals—in this example case, what is best for the students, the course, and curriculum integrity. Taking an "interest-based approach to principled negotiation" (Fisher, Ury, & Patton, 1991) helps both parties focus on the issue rather than the person or on being "right." When we consider the interests of each person, both parties might be surprised to find that their goals are the same. With common goals, each party might be able to put personal issues aside and refocus on solving the problem. Return for a moment to the example of two faculty members disagreeing over specific content to include or exclude in a nursing course. Although faculty members might disagree, if they are truly honest, both will admit their interest in including content vital to student learning, course objectives, and curriculum integrity. In this case, principled negotiation requires each party to focus on the best interest of students rather than argue over whose position is "right."

The Conversation

Critical conversations can be stressful, so prepare by being well-hydrated, well-rested, exercised, and as stress-free as possible. Do some deep breathing exercises or yoga stretches before the meeting. After the meeting begins, use active listening and show genuine interest in your colleague. These are powerful tools in your communication arsenal. Really, truly listening involves attending to the information being communicated and shows genuine concern for your colleague's interest and point of view. Listening and staying focused on your colleague's message can assuage an emotional situation and diffuse negative or hurt feelings. If you find it difficult to listen and concentrate, repeat their words in your head to help you stay focused. Avoid being defensive or judgmental—you might not agree with your colleague's message, but seek to understand it. You also need to avoid interrupting or acting as though you cannot wait to respond and "correct" his or her position or impression. Instead, assume an open and welcoming posture, and affirm his or her message by nodding or issuing brief verbal acknowledgements. Be aware of your nonverbal messages—maintain eye contact, and avoid arm crossing or turning away.

As soon as the conversation begins, each person alternates detailing her or his view and describing her or his perspective of the issue. Each person should adhere to stating objective information and speaking directly and respectfully to the other. Avoid covering up or ignoring your part in the problem or exaggerating the other person's role. The end goal is to find an interest-based resolution, with clear expectations and an agreement regarding who is going to do what by when. If you seek common ground, both give a little, and pursue a compromise, you are more likely to arrive at a win-win solution and ultimately reduce stress levels and improve your working relationship. Be sure to make a plan for a follow-up meeting to evaluate your progress on your efforts to resolve the issue.

During the conversation, I highly suggest using "I" statements and evidence-based models to address the conflict. Using "I" statements helps us open a conversation, but may not necessarily resolve it. In fact, there is no guarantee that any conflict can be resolved—only addressed in a constructive manner. "I" statements help provide clarity about our position, help to preserve or improve relationships rather than making them worse. It is unrealistic to expect an immediate result; however, "I" statements get the conversation started, and provide a step in the right direction to open possibilities for further conversation and negotiating conflict. Conversely, "you" statements are accusatory, blaming, and can trigger defensiveness—these are conversation-stoppers and need to be avoided. Some examples of "I" statements include:

I believe you are saying...

I understand your position to be...

My concern is...

When I'm treated with disrespect...

When I'm not listened to...

When I think I'm not being heard...

I feel unappreciated when...

I'm concerned about...

I feel unimportant when...

I would like...

Could we agree to...

What I'd like to see happen is...

A scenario of a conflicted situation is presented below with a corresponding "I" statement response.

Scenario: *The Case of the Accusing Director*

You recently received a harsh email message from your director summoning you to her office and demanding that you arrive immediately. Reluctantly, you complied, and as you entered the director's office, you sensed an atmosphere of anger and impatience. Without greeting you, the director began blaming you for having a negative influence on other faculty and the nursing program overall. She accused you of raising a controversial issue during a recent faculty meeting with the intent of inciting faculty dissent. The director angrily stated, *"You intentionally asked a derogatory question about curriculum changes which created unnecessary worry among your peers."* You are surprised by the accusation and politely disagree, suggesting that you raised the question in a respectful manner, and it was a genuine attempt to seek clarification. The director vehemently disagreed and instructed you to desist from asking questions in the future. You decide to address the situation.

Addressing the Scenario Using "I" Statements

"It sounds like you're saying that I asked a question in a manner that concerned you. I appreciate your perspective, yet I have a different view. Can we take time for each of us to share our perspectives of what occurred? That way, we can both feel heard and understood."

The next scenario is based on the Caring Feedback Model (Language of Caring, 2016), which includes the following steps:

1. State your positive intent/purpose

2. Describe the specific behavior you noticed or heard about

3. Explain the consequence for you, your team, your patients/students, and the organization

4. Offer a pinch of empathy, and

5. Make a suggestion or request

Scenario: *The Case of Carmen the Nursing Student*

Carmen is consistently late and poorly prepared for her clinical experience. Lately, her clinical performance has deteriorated, patient care has suffered, and her decision-making is suspect. As her clinical instructor, you address these concerns with Carmen.

Addressing the Scenario Using the Caring Feedback Model

Explain your positive purpose: *Carmen, I want to help you become the best nurse you can be.*

Describe specific behavior: *I've noticed that the quality of your work has declined lately and you have been late to clinical for the past three sessions.*

Name the consequence/impact: *I'm concerned about the impact of these behaviors on patient care—not to mention your standing in the course.*

Offer a pinch of empathy: *I realize nursing school can be a stressful experience.*

Make a suggestion/request/expectation: *Nonetheless, it's important to be on time and deliver quality patient care. Let's schedule a meeting to discuss a plan for improvement.*

The next scenario is based on the framework suggested by Casperson (2014), which includes the following elements: When (the triggering event) happened, I felt/believed (feeling/belief) because my (need/interest) is important to me. Would you be willing to (request a doable action)? The scenario demonstrates addressing conflict "in the moment."

Scenario: *The Case of the Gossiping Colleagues*

You are a faculty member in a nursing program. Some faculty members engage in negative gossip and spreading rumors. You believe you have been the target of these behaviors, and one day when you approach the faculty break room, you hear your name mentioned in a derogatory way. As you enter, the faculty fall silent. You decide to address the situation.

Addressing the Scenario Using the Casperson Framework

When I approached the break room, I heard my name mentioned in a negative light. It concerns me because being accepted as a valued member of the team is important to me. In the future, please speak with me directly if you have something to say about me.

The next scenario, which uses the DESC model offered by TeamSTEPPS (Agency for Healthcare Research and Quality [AHRQ], 2016), demonstrates a more planned approach. The DESC steps include D) Describe the specific situation, E) Express your concerns, S) Suggest other alternatives, and C) Consequences stated.

Scenario: *The Case of Conflicted Teaching Team*

You and your colleague, Professor Grey (Terri), are team-teaching a nursing course. You are engaged in a passionate disagreement over specific content to include or exclude in the course. Each of you vehemently disagrees on which subject matter to include, and working together is becoming very stressful. You are actively avoiding Terri and notice she does not reach out to you as often as before. To make matters worse, students are beginning to suffer the consequences of this lack of cooperation. They are becoming confused and frustrated. You realize that something needs to be done to resolve the situation.

Addressing the Scenario Using the DESC Model:

Describe: *Terri, thank you for meeting with me. I'd like to share an observation with you about the course we are co-teaching.*

Express: *I realize that we have differences about our course content, and I'm concerned that this disagreement has begun to impact our relationship as well as our students' ability to learn.*

Suggest: *Because we both genuinely care about our students, it's best if we can work out our differences to provide the best learning experiences for them.*

Consequence: *Let's use our course outcomes/objectives as criteria to address the situation. That way, we're more likely to be successful in reaching agreement.*

Once the conflict is (hopefully) resolved, it is helpful to stop talking about the conflict, find the lesson, forgive it, and move on. If the person you are dealing with is unusually negative and difficult to get along with, be civil, but surround yourself with people who have the qualities you admire and want to emulate. Sometimes this is easier said than done in the workplace. At times we are teamed or partnered with uncivil people. In that case, Pearson and Porath (2009) suggest scheduling shorter meetings, communicating by phone or email, or asking to be reassigned to teams or committees that do not include the uncivil colleague. In addition, avoid meeting with the offender alone, stop attending optional social activities, and work from home as much as possible. Taking these actions is not about sloughing off but about taking care of yourself, and it might mean the difference between your staying and leaving the organization.

If taking a direct approach with your colleague is too difficult or you have tried to work directly with the other person without success, you may need to engage the services of an impartial mediator such as an ombuds, conflict negotiator, or HR representative. You may also consider discussing the situation with your supervisor by asking him or her to explore the situation and assist you in reconciling the problem. If the other person is your supervisor, then you need to rely on the organizational policy for dealing with incivility. Taking such action is not an easy or stress-free decision to make. However, policies exist to protect you from unacceptable behaviors and your employer from costly litigation. If creating a civil workplace is a passion for you, join the teams in your organization that develop and disseminate civility policies (Clark & Ahten, 2011b).

Engaging in critical conversations can be taxing and time-consuming. The nearby sidebar provides several strategies for dealing with negative people. It is also important to take good care of yourself and engage in stress-reducing activities. I was recently chatting with a colleague who was experiencing persistent workplace incivility. I asked him how he dealt with the negativity. He smiled and said, "I conjure up a vision of my wife and children and my beloved family dog, and I feel immediate relief." The conversation reminded me of one of my favorite ways to cope with stressful work situations—I have a number of greeting cards that I have received from family and friends over the years. I keep some of my favorite cards on my desk and select certain ones to cheer me up when needed. At present, I have a lovely anniversary card from my husband propped up on my desk—it features two adorable hummingbirds with sheer love and joy written all over their beautiful, colorful bodies. As silly as it sounds, it works for me.

The card sits alongside a handwritten note that was secretly tucked into my luggage during a recent trip, placed there by our youngest daughter, which reads, "I love you, Mama, have a safe flight and a great trip. I'll miss you." These loved-filled cards and notes take me to a "happy place" where I feel safe, wanted, blessed, and stress-free for just a little while. I also enjoy:

- A bouquet of fresh flowers—grown in our yard and adorning my work space

- Hiking with our furry friends in the cool morning air

- When I worked as a professor, walking across campus and hovering amid the throng of students, especially as classes were changing

- Even better, strolling near the football stadium when the marching band was practicing for home games—the band's excitement and enthusiasm always put me in a better mood

---

STRATEGIES FOR DEALING WITH NEGATIVE PEOPLE

Do not feed into the negativity, and stay detached.

Don't engage every time someone irritates you. Take the high road and walk away.

Surround yourself with positive people.

Imagine being wrapped up tightly in a warm, blue blanket of healing.

Engage in silent, positive self-talk, such as, "This behavior can't affect me unless I let it, and I'm not going to let it."

Maintain healthy boundaries; spend time away from the person as much as possible.

Work from home if your work responsibilities allow.

Show kindness, and pay the negative person a compliment.

Take a walk—get some fresh air.

Conversations With Students

In Chapter 5, I discussed the importance of co-creating, agreeing upon, implementing, and abiding by behavioral classroom and clinical norms. These norms define and guide behavior, help build a community of engagement, and form the basis of seeking common good. Helping students understand how civility applies in real-life situations can be helpful. For example, I have often suggested to my students that they might have an excellent proposal or idea they hope to implement; however, if they demand or insist on implementation without regard for others' points of view, the message is more likely to fall on deaf ears. On the other hand, if they present their case in a respectful and collegial manner and genuinely strive to understand others' perspectives, they stand a greater chance of having the idea implemented. We have also discussed the importance of engaging in respectful interactions and exchanges with colleagues and patients. However, it is not enough to talk about these situations; they must be practiced, discussed, and reinforced.

Faculty must take responsibility for raising civility awareness in students at the very beginning of the students' experience in higher education. We must be very explicit about the behaviors we expect in and out of the classroom and clinical setting. Connelly (2009) recommends that a published Code of Academic Civility be used to stimulate discussion about acceptable behavior, to help students understand that some basic norms and values are transportable from one community to another, and to form the basis for civility. He contends that even though colleges and universities have mission statements and other institutional documents that reinforce civility, faculty members have the responsibility to communicate their content and intent at the beginning of students' college experiences and reinforce their intention throughout their educational experience. Instructional modules are another useful approach for educating students about civility, and they send a clear signal about the importance the institution places on civility.

Putting preventive measures in place can go a long way in reducing the need to deal with incivility. But even with the best-laid plans, you might face times when uncivil behaviors occur. Here are some helpful hints if you experience disruptive student behavior in your classroom. Imagine that a student is talking loudly enough to be heard by everyone in class, making jokes, and clearly distracting other students. First, stay composed, model civility, and do your best to avoid embarrassing the student. Assume that you are being videotaped and that the incident will be uploaded onto YouTube. Because guess what? Someone in the classroom might be taping the events as they unfold with the camera on his or her phone or other device, and even if you're not being taped, assuming you are can help you stay calm and poised. If you have classroom norms, refer to them by making a general statement, such as, "Please remember our agreement to avoid conversations that can get us off track. We have a lot of material to cover, and we can cover it more efficiently if we have everyone's attention."

Remember, it is important to deal with the disruptive behavior immediately or as soon as possible. Ignoring the behavior will likely cause it to continue or increase. Don't take the disruptive behavior personally. It likely has little to do with you, but you must address it. Try a general statement like, "There are several conversations going at the same time, let's all focus on the same topic and work together." If that does not work and the student continues to disrupt the class, you might take a long silent pause, and issue a general word of caution to the entire class: "I am having difficulty concentrating while there is talking; please wait until the break to finish your conversation."

Taking a break is a great stress reliever for you and the class and a good time to meet privately with the offending student. After you and the student are separated from the class and cannot be overheard, use behavioral terms and a nonthreatening approach by saying, "I notice that you seem out of sorts today. What's up?" Listen carefully, and avoid judgment. The student might be forthcoming about the reason for the uncivil behavior—perhaps he or she is stressed out because of a serious family illness or a similar stressful event—or maybe the student has no legitimate reason for the bad behavior. In either case, discuss your observations frankly and honestly, identify options, and, if necessary, ask the student to leave for the day and connect him or her to support services.

When Disruptive Behavior Becomes Threatening

In some instances, simply talking with a student might be insufficient, ineffective, or inadequate to the scope of what the situation calls for. If a student's behavior becomes threatening, once again, remain as calm as possible, but act swiftly and firmly. Even if you have just given a break, give another one. This act alone might help calm the situation. Then ask the offending student to leave class (or clinical) for the remainder of the day. If the student refuses to leave, call campus (or hospital) security to help escort the student from class or clinical. If you perceive that you or others are in imminent danger, call 911 or contact Campus Police immediately. Contact your department chairperson or immediate supervisor as soon as possible, and refer the student to university Student Services so the policies for disruptive student behavior can be implemented.

You may be asked to meet with the student to address the offending behavior. Behaviors such as profane language, making threats, and issuing harassing or intimidating comments require further intervention. These situations necessitate meeting privately with the student and implementing best practices for addressing threatening behaviors:

- Document observations (be objective and precise).

- Meet during business hours, use a conference room, and sit closest to the door.

- Inform at least one other faculty member/supervisor about the meeting; have him/her available in the surrounding area.

- Don't place items on the table that can be used as weapons of opportunity.

- Discuss your observations frankly and honestly.

- Outline the expected behaviors, options, and resources.

- Issue consequences/sanctions (refer to Code of Conduct and other policies and procedures).

- Clarify your capacity to help—refer to experts (Student Services).

SIGNS OF BEHAVIORAL ESCALATION

Though no specific profile for students who might demonstrate or carry out threatening or violent behaviors exists, we must all be alert for signs of disruptive behaviors that might potentially occur or escalate. Consider whether the student might be under the influence of drugs or alcohol, whether he or she is suffering from a mental illness, or whether the quality of his or her assignments has suddenly declined or they contain veiled or direct threats. Students might write or say something like, "You're going to be sorry for the grade you issued," or, "You just wait—I know where you live, and I can find you." In these situations, mandatory reporting is required.

Students Starting the Conversation

Faculty can use the same framework described earlier in this chapter to help students learn and rehearse critical conversations in classroom and clinical settings. At some point in a student's education, he or she might want to discuss uncivil situations encountered with other students, faculty, nurses in practice, or administrators. During the reflecting and probing phase, and before committing to the conversation, students should thoughtfully reflect on their own behaviors, consider the intent and context of the event, and, as objectively as possible, ponder their potential contributions to the situation. If, after careful reflection, the student still believes that he or she has been treated disrespectfully, he or she can use the framework covered earlier in the chapter to discuss the interaction with the offender. If a student is apprehensive about a face-to-face meeting, sending a polite email asking for clarification (and/or a meeting) can be helpful. An exemplar is provided in the nearby sidebar.

EXAMPLE STUDENT-TO-FACULTY EMAIL

Dear Professor Green,

I would like to meet with you at your earliest convenience to discuss important issues related to our clinical experience. Given your busy schedule, and the importance of this request, I have provided several dates/times below for your consideration [then list 3–4 dates/times]. Please let me know which date/time works best for you and where you would like to meet. I look forward to hearing from you soon.

Respectfully,
Dana Smith, NU 333

However, though an email message can help get the conversation started, having an in-person meeting can be empowering and excellent practice for similar encounters students might face throughout their career. Taking a direct and honest route is clearly the best strategy, but it takes fortitude and practice, practice, practice.

Email messaging has changed the way we communicate and conduct business. Though it is a speedy, swift, and efficient way to send and receive information, it has also affected the manner in which we express our thoughts and feelings and how we interpret communications and expressions of others. Unfortunately, email does not allow us to see the verbal and nonverbal messages that might otherwise be conveyed in face-to-face communication. Some of the problems with email communication are included in the accompanying sidebar.

THE DOWNSIDES OF EMAIL MESSAGING

The intent of the email message may be misinterpreted.

The message might be sent before the message is fully crafted.

The message might be sent or forwarded to the wrong person.

The message might be "blind copied" to others without your knowledge.

The message might be altered to suit the whim of the sender.

The emotional content of the message might be misunderstood or misrepresented.

The lack of nonverbal cues (facial expressions, inflection, and body language) might add to misinterpretation.

Nursing students also need communication skills to function effectively as confident, assertive team members. Facilitating critical conversations begins with and must continue throughout a student's nursing education. Teaching our students about the importance of communication requires more than discussion—it requires simulating, demonstrating, practicing, and rehearsing these fundamental skills over and over again (Clark & Ahten, 2010). Because nursing education and practice are inextricably linked, conversations about incivility must begin early in a student's education. These conversations must be multilayered and progress sequentially throughout the students' education. Post-clinical debriefings and assignments incorporating self-reflection can be used to bring attention to uncivil incidents and how to successfully address them. This allows students a safe place to relate their experiences, share their impressions, receive constructive feedback, and learn appropriate ways of managing such situations (Clark & Ahten, 2010).

Simulations can be used to create uncivil, high-anxiety scenarios that give students a safe place to make mistakes, practice conflict-resolution skills, and observe firsthand how a gesture or word choice can influence the outcome of a situation. Students in more senior courses can examine incivility in broader context, such as managing employee conflict, understanding and implementing organizational civility policies, establishing a culture of civility within an organization, and understanding how managers' attitudes and behaviors influence the actions of their staff. Engaging students in these meaningful, critical conversations can go a long way in promoting personal and organizational civility. In Chapter 10, I describe a civility/incivility exercise for students in great detail.

Emotions and Effective Communication

Emotions play an important role in the way we communicate with others; how we feel about and experience a situation affects how we deal with it. Emotions influence how we understand and react to others, including uncivil encounters, and ultimately how we manage them. When we are out of touch with our emotions, suppress our feelings, or refuse to acknowledge them, communication becomes much more difficult. When we avoid dealing with situations that bother us, we can become frustrated, angry, or withdrawn. Becoming aware of and understanding our emotions enhance our ability to effectively communicate, problem-solve, resolve conflicts, and work more collaboratively with others.

Emotional intelligence (EI) is the ability to perceive and express emotions, to use emotions to facilitate thinking, to understand and reason with emotions, and to manage emotions effectively within oneself and in relationships with others (Mayer, Salovey, & Caruso, 2000). Simply put, EI is the ability to understand our emotions and the emotions of others and to use this understanding to interact collaboratively with others. People who exhibit emotional awareness and self-control can handle conflicting situations more effectively. Freshman and Rubino (2002) describe five core areas of EI: self-awareness, self-regulation, self-motivation, social awareness, and social skills. The authors conclude that EI is a core competency for healthcare professionals and that only a few progressive healthcare facilities have recognized the value of EI training and incorporated programs that emphasize its principles into their organizations. Table 8.1 is a summary of the components and definitions of EI (Freshman & Rubino, 2002).

Table 8.1 COMPONENTS AND DEFINITIONS OF EMOTIONAL INTELLIGENCE

COMPONENT	DEFINITION
Self-awareness	A deep understanding of one's emotions, strengths, weaknesses, needs, and drives
Self-regulation	A propensity for reflection, ability to adapt to changes, saying no to impulsive urges
Self-motivation	Driven to achieve and being passionate about one's profession and enjoying challenges
Social awareness	Thoughtfully considering others' feelings when acting
Social skills	Moving people in the desired direction

EI is closely related to emotional awareness, which involves the ability to recognize and label your emotions and to express and manage them without becoming overwhelmed. It means knowing what we are feeling and why we feel the way we do and then acting with diplomacy and skill. Emotional awareness is an ability we can learn and, with practice, master. Emotional awareness helps us empathize with others, discover what is really bothering us, communicate more clearly, and build collegial relationships. The goal of effective communication is to find a healthy balance between intellect and emotion, and between thinking and feeling. Because emotions are the connective tissue that links us together, we do not want to lose control of them—but instead want to manage them to enjoy more satisfying relationships.

Some of us worry about being becoming too emotional, losing control, or appearing weak or vulnerable if we engage in a critical conversation. However, when emotions are handled appropriately and stress is well-managed, we can realize several positive outcomes, including improved teamwork, stronger interpersonal relationships, greater productivity, and healthier work environments. On the other hand, the cost of suppressing emotions and feelings can cause physical and psychological distress, decreased motivation, and a lower level of job satisfaction. Fortunately, we can improve our level of EI and emotional awareness.

Although some aspects of EI cannot be tested or measured, some assessments can give you an idea of your EI skills. In the past, I have assigned readings on the topic of EI to my nursing students and had them complete a free online assessment at www.queendom.com/tests/iq/emotional_iq_r2_access.html. After students completed the EI assessment, I asked them to respond to a set of questions, including:

1. Please summarize your EI results by sharing only what you are comfortable sharing.

2. Describe what you learned about yourself after completing the EI assessment.

3. Which aspects of your EI assessment are most significant to you? Explain.

4. Based on what you have learned from your EI assessment, what techniques might you use in a situation where you had to curb your natural tendencies or behaviors? For example, if you are uncomfortable with conflict, what could you do in situations where you know conflict will occur?

5. How is knowing your EI assessment related to becoming an effective nurse and leader? Explain your position.

Learning more about ourselves and the way we commonly respond in certain situations can give us greater confidence in communicating with others. When we identify and address our areas for growth and improvement (as well as our strengths), we increase our ability to interact with civility. However, just because we act in a civil manner does not guarantee that others will reciprocate. Nonetheless, our individual civil acts contribute to the construction and maintenance of a *civility infrastructure* that benefits all (Maxey, 2011, p. 37). Similarly, Forni (2008) encourages us to follow eight rules for a civil life (see the accompanying sidebar).

Despite our best efforts to manage our stress levels and to live a civil life, strong emotions can be triggered with little warning or predictability. It would be great if we could hurry and get a massage or go for a quick run—or in my case, don my boxing gloves and kick and punch some heavy bags—but often we need to respond quickly and implement "ready-to-use" skills as the stressful situation occurs. This requires a combination of managing feeling and thinking skills to make sound decisions. Benegbi

(2012) recommends seven steps to achieving *calm confidence*—an ability to adjust immediately in any given situation. Her techniques for controlling emotions and reactions more naturally are summarized in the nearby sidebar.

DR. FORNI'S EIGHT RULES FOR A CIVIL LIFE

1. *Slow down and be present in your life.*

2. *Listen to the voice of empathy.*

3. *Keep a positive attitude.*

4. *Respect others and grant them plenty of validation.*

5. *Disagree graciously and refrain from arguing.*

6. *Get to know the people around you.*

7. *Pay attention to the small things.*

8. *Ask, don't tell.*

SEVEN STEPS TO ACHIEVING CALM CONFIDENCE

Breathe: *Take long, slow, deep breaths in and out through your nose. Continue breathing as you bring your hands together as if you are about to clap them, palms pressed together in front of you, relaxed. This helps induce a neutral state to assess the situation from a clear perspective.*

Smile: *Changing your projection and smiling helps you change your mood, energy, and feelings.*

Drink a glass of water *to shift energy and balance the system.*

Repeat positive affirmations *to adjust your thinking—such as "I am strong." "I am calm."*

Adjust your posture: *Straighten your spine, relax your shoulders, lift your chest, bring your chin in a little, and breathe. This helps remove blocked energy and allows energy to flow.*

Take a 5-minute break: Go to a quiet place where you can take several deep breaths.

Tune into the potential within you: Breathe, tell yourself to relax, and be guided by the teacher within. Ask for guidance and be open to a different perspective.

(Benegbi, 2012)

Practicing these calm-confidence strategies and implementing the self-care and stress-reducing strategies described in Chapter 11 can be very helpful, yet at times, an immediate, direct response is needed to acknowledge the uncivil behavior without offering excuses or opinions. When an insult is hurled your way, here are a few thoughts to consider. First, pause and take a moment to reflect on the person's intent. It does not matter if it is true or not; what matters is the perceived intent. Knowing this will help you respond in an effective manner. If you determine that the person is deliberately trying to insult you, you may simply choose to ignore the comment and walk away, indicating that the comment is so ridiculous that it is not worth your time or energy.

But what if you want to stick up for yourself (especially if insulting you has become a pattern with this individual)? I suggest that you stay poised and composed and say something like, "Your comment sounded like an insult to me. I hope that wasn't your intent." And, then calmly walk away. Or let's suppose you are repeatedly criticized by a colleague for not "pulling your weight"—you can say, "When I'm criticized about the pace of my work, it distracts me from preparing classes and meeting with students. Please avoid making these comments so that I can focus on my work responsibilities." Confronting an uncivil coworker can be challenging, but it often puts an end to the problem by directly addressing the offensive behavior.

Finishing Touches

Changing the culture means changing our individual and collective conversations. Dealing with incivility takes personal courage and requires each of us to take action to stop uncivil behavior. Confronting an uncivil individual can be challenging, but it often puts an end to the problem by directly addressing the offensive behavior. Taking care of our mind and body and reducing stress can pay vast dividends for our emotional and physical health. Learning to effectively communicate and engage in critical conversations must be mindful and intentional. It takes all of us to reverse the insidious nature and related consequences of incivility to ultimately create a sustained culture of civility.

CIVILITY TIP

Next time you feel compelled to return or send an unpleasant email message, take a deep breath, reconsider, and wait at least 24 hours before responding. Then, craft the message, reread it several times, and if it fails to convey the message you want to express, hit the Delete key. However, if the message meets the four-way ethical criteria provided by Rotary International— meaning the message is truthful, fair, builds goodwill and better friendships, and is beneficial to all concerned—then by all means, hit the Send key.

Chapter 9

The First Day of Class: Co-Creating a Positive Learning Environment

The issues of character and civility are not merely esoteric or an add-on to the curriculum, like driver's education. They are central to our mission and to our very survival as an institution and a society. –Paul D. Houston (Center for Empowered Leadership)

This chapter discusses:

- Preventing uncivil behavior in the classroom
- Leveraging the first day of class
- Crafting your teaching philosophy
- Co-creating norms of behavior

Framework for Primary Prevention

I fervently believe that the greater effort we make on the first day of class to prevent uncivil and disruptive behavior from occurring, the better it is for everyone. This investment can pay lasting dividends over the course of the academic term and beyond. I ascribe to a primary prevention approach to addressing incivility. Dealing with the least disruptive behaviors and preventing them from occurring in the first place contributes to a safe, civil learning environment focused on student and faculty success.

The Public Health Approach to Violence Prevention Model used by the national Centers for Disease Control and Prevention (Dalhberg & Krug, 2002) provides a useful structure to frame the problem of incivility in nursing education (see Figure 9.1). The model illustrates a systematic process that involves four steps:

1. Defining the problem

2. Identifying risk and protective factors

3. Developing and testing prevention strategies

4. Ensuring widespread adoption

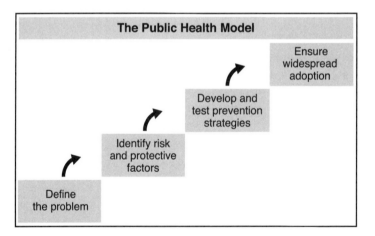

FIGURE 9.1

Public Health Approach to Violence Prevention Model (Centers for Disease Control and Prevention).

The first step in preventing incivility and potential violence is to understand it and to identify the factors that contribute to it. Some of the factors contributing to incivility in nursing education include high stress levels; overwork and overextension with family, work, and school demands; exposure to uncivil and bullying behaviors; inability to effectively communicate and negotiate conflict; and an imbalance of power (Clark, 2008a; Clark, Olender, Cardoni, & Kenski, 2011).

The second step of the prevention model identifies risks and protective factors. Potential risks associated with student incivility include stress due to burnout from demanding workloads, perceived competition in a high-stakes academic environment, and an intense competition for grades and scholarships (Clark, 2008a). Risks associated with faculty incivility include dealing with heavy workloads and workload inequity, maintaining clinical competence, addressing advancement issues, dealing with a lack of administrative support, and keeping pace with technology (Clark, 2013; Clark & Springer, 2010). We need to use prevention strategies to address these risk factors to inhibit disruptive behaviors from escalating into more dangerous situations. I describe strategies and preventive measures in detail later in this chapter.

The third step of the prevention model involves developing and testing prevention strategies. The strategies included in this chapter include setting a positive tone, reviewing key "talking points" contained in the course syllabus, incorporating behavioral objectives, sharing teaching philosophies, co-creating classroom and clinical norms, and discussing the major concepts related to the course and/or curriculum (which I often refer to as "super threads"—the foundational elements of the course).

The final step of the prevention model calls for widespread adoption of effective strategies to prevent incivility and possible violence. This chapter provides nursing faculty with several evidence-based, ready-to-use strategies to foster a safer learning environment and to promote a culture of civility in nursing education.

The Imperative for Civility, Professionalism, and Ethical Practice in Nursing

All nurses (including nursing faculty and students) have an ethical responsibility to foster healthy workplaces and to promote an atmosphere of dignity, professionalism, and respect. As I mentioned in Chapter 2, in every Gallup poll since 1999 (except 2001 following the 9/11 attacks, when first responders were rated higher), Americans have rated nurses highest on honesty and ethical standards (Gallup. (2016). Honesty/ ethics in professions. Retrieved from http://www.gallup.com/poll/1654/ honesty-ethics-professions.aspx). As nurses, we must behave in ways that merit this impressive distinction. The International Council of Nurses (ICN) *Code of Ethics for Nurses* (2012), the American Nurses Association (ANA) *Code of Ethics for Nurses with Interpretive Statements* (2015a), and other important professional documents and statements provide a firm foundation for implementing teaching strategies and curricula to foster healthy work environments and to ensure the delivery of safe, quality patient care.

For years, I have been designing and implementing an evidence-based approach to integrate the concepts of civility, professionalism, and ethical practice into nursing curricula. This evidence-based approach is an effective way to incorporate these essential concepts without creating an additional burden for faculty. Instead of adding to an already jam-packed curriculum, this integrated approach is intended to be flexible and complement student learning outcomes focused on concepts that already exist in nearly every nursing curriculum. Think about it: The concepts of civility, professionalism, and ethics are foundational to all nursing education curricula. Therefore, rather than adding to a curriculum, faculty are enhancing what they are already doing to amplify these concepts. For more detail, see Clark (Clark, 2017).

Let's begin with definitions. Although the concepts of civility, professionalism, and ethical practice are interrelated, I would like to define each one separately to provide a deeper understanding of each individual concept. First, *civility* includes honoring differences, discussing them robustly, and treating one another with dignity, honor, and respect (Emry & Holmes, 2005; Guinness, 2008). A concept analysis of civility noted in Chapter 1 found that being civil requires time, presence, engagement, an authentic respect for others, and intention to seek common ground (Clark & Carnosso, 2008).

DeLesky (2013) defines *professionalism* as the "assimilation of nursing skills and knowledge integrated with dignity and respect for all human beings, incorporating the assumptions and values of the profession while maintaining accountability and self-awareness" (p. 359). According to Crigger and Godfrey (2014), *professional identity* in nursing refers to an individual's perception of himself or herself and the fulfillment of responsibilities toward society, recipients of care, other professionals, and to himself or herself. This process is influenced by characteristics, norms, and values of the nursing discipline resulting in an individual thinking, acting, and feeling like a nurse.

According to the ANA (2015a), *ethical practice* is a "promise that nurses are doing their best to provide care for their patients and their communities and are supporting each other in the process so that all nurses can fulfill their ethical and professional obligations" (p. 40). *Respect for persons* is an ethical principle and an element of professionalism which maintains that "human beings have an unconditional moral worth that requires us to treat each individual person with value, dignity, and respect" (Giddons, 2013, p. 389). When these interconnected, interrelated concepts are lacking or underdeveloped, the potential for incivility increases. On the other hand, when civility, professionalism, and ethical practice are integrated into nursing curricula, the potential for fostering safe, civil workplaces is heightened.

Successful integration of these key concepts into nursing curricula requires implementing a variety of evidence-based interventions and active learning strategies. Nurse educators must equip themselves with strategies to prepare the next generation of nurses to create positive change, foster healthy work environments, and ensure safe patient care. An integrated, evidence-based curricular approach is introduced in the following sections.

In Chapters 2 and 5, I highlighted the important need for all institutions of higher learning to create and widely disseminate clearly articulated vision, mission, and shared values statements to all members of the campus community with an intentional focus on academic citizenship and civility. These statements—which include a brief description of civility, an explanation of the importance of respecting each person's dignity, and a list of institutional values that are shared with all members of the campus community—need to be emphasized during new-student orientation to the campus. New-student orientation to the nursing program reinforces adherence to the foundational statements and underscores the importance of civility, professionalism, socialization to the profession, and ethical practice.

The emphasis on these key concepts is not limited to new student orientation, and must be integrated throughout the curriculum over the duration of the students' nursing education experience. This integration may be accomplished by engaging students in specific activities and exercises such as having them complete the Civility Index for Students (Chapter 10) to assess their perceptions of respectful interactions and civility acumen; incorporating role-play, simulation, and unfolding case studies focused on civility, professionalism, and ethical practice into various classes; facilitating professional workshops and journal clubs; and involving students in other program activities that stress the importance of these key concepts. Examples are detailed in the next chapter.

Faculty as Positive Role Models

You get only one chance to make a first impression.

Being a positive, professional role model and setting the best example we can for students, coworkers, and practice partners is one of the most formidable tools in the civility toolbox. First impressions matter and are often made at lightning speed. When students meet faculty for the first time, they register myriad impressions, and often these impressions are lasting ones. Therefore, it is important to consider how we present, interact, communicate, and treat others. I have developed a Civility Index for Faculty to use as a reflective exercise to measure perceptions of faculty civility. The index is designed to raise awareness and determine strengths and opportunities for civility improvement. The index, which is shown nearby, may be completed as an individual self-reflection exercise, or co-completed with a colleague to garner another perspective of one's civility acumen.

CIVILITY INDEX FOR FACULTY

To complete the index, consider the 20 statements listed below. Read each statement carefully and select the response that most accurately represents the frequency of each behavior by asking yourself how often do I (OR how often do my coworkers):
(1) Never (2) Rarely (3) Sometimes (4) Usually (5) Always

Regard students as adult learners and expect them to succeed	1	2	3	4	5
Role-model civility, professionalism, and respectful discourse	1	2	3	4	5
Believe students add value and meaning to the educational experience	1	2	3	4	5
Communicate respectfully (by email, telephone, face-to-face) and really listen	1	2	3	4	5
Avoid gossip and making sarcastic or demeaning comments about students	1	2	3	4	5
Come to class prepared and use evidence-based teaching/learning strategies	1	2	3	4	5
Use respectful language (avoid racial, ethnic, sexual, gender, religiously biased terms)	1	2	3	4	5
Encourage other faculty to observe and provide feedback on my teaching methods	1	2	3	4	5
Co-create and abide by classroom and clinical norms	1	2	3	4	5
Address disruptive student behaviors and promote a safe, civil learning environment	1	2	3	4	5
Take personal responsibility and stand accountable for my actions	1	2	3	4	5
Avoid reprimanding the entire class for one student's misbehavior	1	2	3	4	5
Utilize objective grading criteria and assignment rubrics	1	2	3	4	5
Avoid exerting superiority or position over students (threatening to fail them)	1	2	3	4	5
Keep office hours, return emails, and maintain availability outside of class	1	2	3	4	5
Uphold the vision, mission, and values of my organization	1	2	3	4	5
Listen to and incorporate constructive feedback from students	1	2	3	4	5
Demonstrate an openness to other points of view	1	2	3	4	5
Include, welcome, encourage, and mentor students	1	2	3	4	5
Apologize and mean it when the situation calls for it	1	2	3	4	5

Scoring the Civility Index: Add up the number of 1–5 responses to determine your civility score

90–100—Very civil	60–69—Minimally civil
80–89—Civil	50–59—Uncivil
70–79—Moderately civil	Less than 50—Very uncivil

The First Day of Class: Greetings, Introductions, and Name Tents

Nursing faculty can implement several strategies prior to and during the first day of class to set a positive tone for a successful academic term. Professional role-modeling and demonstrating civility are great ways to begin. Consider implementing some of the following strategies. One to two weeks before classes start, send a "welcoming" email message to students, briefing them on the agenda for the first day—include a greeting, where class will meet and when class begins, materials needed for class, and the day's objectives. Include the syllabus and course calendar, and suggest that students review both before attending class. Next, arrive early on the first day of class (and every day after) to set up your classroom and teaching-learning materials to be ready to greet students as they come through the door.

When I meet my students on the first day, I welcome them by introducing myself, asking their names, and handing each student a colorful, large (blank) index card. It is fun to watch students take the card and ask or wonder about the card's purpose. I realize I have accomplished what I hoped—first, to heighten curiosity and, second, to connect with each student using a "high-touch teaching strategy." Later in class, students will discover the purpose of the index card and will use them to create name tents; this process is discussed later in this chapter.

When students are assembled and seated, I officially start class. After a more formal welcome and a review of the day's objectives, I begin class with student introductions. My introduction will follow theirs. Because I have large classes (approximately 75 students per class), I need to keep introductions brief, but meaningful. Students can introduce themselves very quickly, and interesting information can be gleaned from each one by utilizing fill-in-the-blank questions. For example, my students take turns introducing themselves by standing, stating their first and last name, and completing a fill-in-the-blank question provided on a PowerPoint slide or written on the white board. For example, I have asked students to respond to the following fill-in-the-blank question: "If I could change the world, I would _____ (fill in the blank)."

Other times I have used a question directly related to the course that I am teaching. For example, when teaching a behavioral health course, I might ask the following fill-in-the-blank question: "When I hear the term mental illness, I think _____ (fill in the blank)."

These probing questions are excellent vehicles to introduce (or re-introduce in a fresh way) students to one another and to the faculty and to provide a window into how students think and what each believes about a particular and course-relevant topic. This engaging, and often amusing, exercise can help us learn a little bit about our students' worldviews and life perspectives on the first day.

If the size of your class is particularly large or if you are concerned that having students introduce themselves individually may hold little interest for other students, it may be more effective to have students form dyads or small groups, have them introduce themselves to one another, and then have students take turns introducing their classmates to the class at large. In either case, this is a good time to check the accuracy of the the enrollment roster—in my classes, I often asked a student to volunteer to manage the class roster so that I could be more attentive as students introduced themselves and/or each other. Introductions are also a good time to have students create their name tents (see Figure 9.2).

Students are more motivated and feel valued by teachers who know their names. There are several strategies for getting to know our students by name. One of my favorite methods is to use name tents. Prior to introductions, I describe the process and purpose for name tents, so that students can create them during introductions. I ask students to fold their large index cards lengthwise, and using the magic markers that I have provided, to write their preferred name on both sides of the index card. If feasible, you can arrange the students in a manner (such as semicircles) that allows for the name tents to be visible to all class participants. This technique builds respect, collegiality, and an *esprit de corps* among faculty and students. Name tents help all of us learn each student's name quickly and remove the embarrassment of forgetting a student's name—or worse, addressing them by pointing or using impersonal statements. Students bring their name tents to each class meeting. Visitors and guest speakers appreciate them and value being able to call students by name. However, we as faculty need to be transparent and explain to students why we do what we do—and in the case of name tents, the primary reason for using them is to show respect by getting to know students by name and recognizing the uniqueness that each student brings to the learning environment.

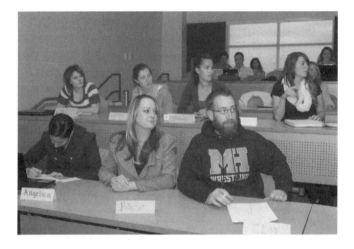

FIGURE 9.2
Students with name tents.

Another way to learn students' names is to have them state their name each time they speak or interact with the class. This process can be continued until everyone feels they know each person in the class. In my classes, I downloaded a photo of each student to correspond with the information included on the class roster. I took time to review the photos and corresponding names and placed them on my desk as I evaluated and graded assignments. Putting a face to a name helped accelerate learning my students' names. Students may be asked to select a seat of their choice and continue using the seat throughout the term so that a seating chart can be created. If your class is small, you can make appointments with each student during the first 1 or 2 weeks of class to get to know them better. However you decide to learn your students' names, be honest and let them know that getting to know their names is important to you, but that it may take a bit of time (particularly in large classes). After students have completed their introductions and created their name tents, I introduce myself, an explicit example of role-modeling politeness and civility by having others go first.

The Power of the Course Syllabus

The course syllabus is an excellent tool to assist faculty both with facilitating classroom discussion about expected goals, objectives, and important policies and guidelines and with establishing behavioral norms. Faculty need to devote as much time as necessary on the first day of class to review the syllabus, to describe teaching philosophies, to discuss the role of civil discourse, and to clarify assignments and expected behaviors. An ambiguous or poorly constructed syllabus can contribute to student resentment and anger, whereas a well-developed and thoughtfully discussed syllabus can be a catalyst for civility and co-creating classroom and clinical norms (Clark, 2009).

The course syllabus is a "contract" with students and can be used as a guide to discuss what we expect to accomplish together as faculty and students throughout the course of the term. Syllabi can include a number of important topics, links, and talking points, which serve as a foundation for co-creating behavioral norms and creating and sustaining a civil, safe learning environment.

Faculty need to perform a comprehensive review of the syllabus on the first day of class. Some faculty like to have students review the course syllabus on their own prior to the beginning of classes, believing it will save time and allow for other "more important" content to be covered. This approach might be valid; however, I believe the syllabus is so important, and its review so helpful, that I highly suggest you make it a part of the first day of class. I've already mentioned that you can include web links that provide talking points for creating a safe, civil teaching-learning environment, but beyond that a good syllabus can shrink-wrap many important topics and policies, providing key information as short, pithy statements. For example, the program's conflict-negotiation policy can be summarized briefly and a link inserted into the syllabus. Faculty can use this talking point to facilitate an intentional conversation with students about the policy and its implementation. This dialogue gets to the heart of the matter—to help students learn the key elements of conflict negotiation, how the process works in the school of nursing, and how they might use it if a conflict arises with another student or a faculty member. Walking through the steps of the conflict-negotiation process equips students with helpful information to deal directly with conflict in the academic setting and prepares them to address conflicts that might occur in the practice setting. I encourage students to come to me directly if they experience a conflict with me—that way, we can work together to successfully resolve the issue. My goal is to role-model transparency, professionalism, and successful conflict-negotiation processes. By engaging students in the discussion points regarding the syllabus, I have had extremely few conflicts; and in the rare circumstance when a conflict arose, by meeting and talking directly with one another, we have arrived at a mutually acceptable solution.

Another talking point example includes the policy for academic dishonesty and plagiarism. Again, including a link to the policy is helpful, but discussing the policy and sharing examples of academic dishonesty, such as plagiarizing a paper or cheating on exams, are necessary. Many students are unclear about the definition and types of academic dishonesty, so give examples, discuss the consequences of academic dishonesty, and most importantly, describe how to achieve academic honesty. Many nursing programs use a template whereby all faculty members include various policy links and definitions in the course syllabus, including definitions of academic dishonesty, cheating, and plagiarizing.

Academic Dishonesty, Cheating, and Plagiarism

Our institutional definitions read as follows:

- *Academic dishonesty* can include cheating, plagiarism, or other forms of academic dishonesty. All assignments submitted by a student must represent her/his own ideas, concepts, and current understanding or must cite the original source. Attempts to violate the academic integrity of an assignment do not have to be successful to be considered academic dishonesty.

- *Cheating* includes any action where an individual or group either carries out or attempts to carry out dishonest work and/or where an individual or group either assists or attempts to assist an individual or group to carry out dishonest work. If students are uncertain whether an action constitutes cheating, they have a responsibility to ask the faculty member for the course for clarification.

- *Plagiarism* at its most basic level means to steal someone else's words, composition, research, and/or ideas. Plagiarism is both cheating and theft. Given the seriousness of this offense, students have a responsibility to understand its meaning and implications for the academic community.

After reviewing the definitions, we then discuss examples of academic dishonesty and ways to prevent them. Examples of plagiarism include using another person's work, published or unpublished, without clearly quoting, citing, or fully acknowledging the work or using materials prepared by a person or agency engaged in the selling of term papers or other academic materials. We also review Lipson's (2004) three principles to avoid academic dishonesty:

- When you say you did the work, you actually did it.

- When you rely on someone else's work, you cite it. When you use their words, you quote them fully and accurately—and cite them.

- When you present research materials, you present them fairly and truthfully.

Academic dishonesty is not a new phenomenon in higher education; however, digital technology has expanded the opportunities and possibilities for engaging in such practices, because information is free and only a click away (Levine & Dean, 2012). According to senior student affairs officers, a growing number of students don't understand that plagiarism is wrong because many traditional-age students have grown up collaborating with friends online and sharing content they find on the Internet. These same student affairs officers recommend that syllabi be used to address rules of conduct including issues related to academic dishonesty (Levine & Dean, 2012). As faculty, we must be very clear with students; if they have any questions regarding an assignment and its level of academic honesty or dishonesty, they need to contact faculty or other university resources for assistance.

Other talking points might include the academic code of conduct, professional standards and behaviors, codes of ethics, and proper use of social networking and online etiquette. For example, we need to discuss the purpose and aspects of the protocol for social networking in the nursing programs, both to inform students about the appropriate use of online social-networking sites as it relates to professional conduct expected of nursing students and to reinforce the use of online social-networking postings in accordance with codes of conduct and standards of professional behavior. Nursing students are encouraged to read the "White Paper: A Nurse's Guide to the Use of Social Media" published by the National Council of State Boards of Nursing (2011). Because some students are ill-informed about the use of social networking in nursing, they find that the white paper is a rich and excellent resource.

The syllabus should also contain clear learning objectives and associated assignments (with rationale for each) and rubrics for grading course assignments and projects. In addition to the academic objectives (aka competencies, outcomes) required in all courses, each course should include a behavioral objective. Behavioral objectives reinforce student accountability for the professional nursing role and are based on nursing standards of care and professional performance (ANA, 2015c). At times, a student might be meeting the academic objectives of the course, might even be getting an "A" in the class; however, if the student is acting in an unprofessional manner inconsistent with the behavioral course objective, the student might still fail the course if the behavioral objective remains unmet.

Here are two examples of behavioral objectives:

- Demonstrates accountability for one's own personal and professional conduct, which reflect the standards, values, and ethical behaviors of the profession.

- Models the professional nursing role, based on acceptable standards of practice and ethical principles, including being accountable for one's personal and professional behaviors and development.

A behavioral objective coupled with a direct faculty-student conversation is a powerful combination for improving behavior expected of a nursing student and a professional nurse. I am a big fan of Dr. Susan Luparell's approach to engaging students on the topic of behavioral objectives (S. Luparell, personal communication). On the first day of class, Luparell asks her students for a show of hands in response to the question, "How many of you [students] aspire to become marginal or mediocre nurses?" Of course, no one raises a hand. Then she asks, "How many of you aspire to become highly proficient and expert nurses?" In this case, all students raise their hand. Then she adds, "This is great news, because as your teacher, there might come a time when I need to give you helpful feedback on how you can become a highly proficient and expert nurse. If that happens, I will remind you of our agreement today, so the feedback might be more readily received." This brilliant strategy sets the stage for future meetings where faculty might need to address performance or academic issues with students.

Bringing Our Teaching Philosophies Into the Light

Stephen Brookfield (1990) defines a *teaching philosophy* as a personal vision of teaching, including critical rationale and purpose(s) for teaching. Teaching philosophies represent ideas, beliefs, and assumptions about teaching, teaching strategies, methods and objectives, ways to put these beliefs and strategies into practice, and goals for student learning. Brookfield notes that a teaching philosophy can be used as an organizing vision—a clear picture of why you teach, and for what pedagogical purposes—to describe the effect we hope to have on students and on their learning. The structure and formatting of teaching philosophies vary, but most statements are personal and reflective, well-developed and concise, written using first-person narrative, and crafted with the intended audience in mind. They provide a unique description of our perspective on teaching and our professional commitment to learners.

Faculty can develop both individual and team teaching philosophies. In nursing education, much of the teaching is done in teams. Sharing our team and individual teaching philosophies with students and being clear and explicit about our values and beliefs help create a safe, civil learning environment. When students understand our views, methods, and rationale, they are more likely to feel engaged in and part of the learning process.

As a nursing professor, my primary teaching responsibilities included teaching and coordinating the nursing leadership courses in the prelicensure bachelor of science program in the school of nursing. I was tasked with coordinating a team of approximately seven faculty members—all of whom teach and facilitate student projects in the clinical portion of our leadership course. Team membership might ebb and flow; however, the nucleus of our team remained stable for many years. Several years ago, our teaching team met for a day-long, off-campus retreat to develop and agree upon our team teaching philosophy for the nursing leadership clinical course. We used a variation of the "visioning" process detailed in Chapter 5 (Latham, 1995) to create our vision, mission, and philosophy statements. The statements are powerful assertions to share with students, community partners, and one another. Our goal was to demonstrate how the faculty teaching team is united in helping students meet the course objectives. Though each clinical group might meet the course objectives in varying ways, students realize that the faculty shares a common vision, mission, and philosophy to accomplish those objectives. Our philosophical statements emphasize professionalism, inclusion, a student-centered approach to teaching and learning, commitment to individual and collective achievement, and the expectation of civility in all interactions. Each academic year, our faculty teaching team reviewed, revised (if needed), and reaffirmed our philosophical statements. They were also published in our clinical course syllabus and shared and reinforced with students and community partners (preceptors) on the first day of classes and beyond. Our teaching team vision, mission, and philosophy are provided in the nearby sidebar.

NURSING LEADERSHIP AND MANAGEMENT
TEACHING TEAM VISION, MISSION, AND
PHILOSOPHY

Vision

To develop ethical, principled nurses who possess leadership and management skills to effect meaningful change in a variety of healthcare settings and organizations.

Mission

To practice professionalism, inclusion, collaboration, and civility through open dialogue, civil discourse, engagement, and essential conversation to promote learning, professional growth, and development.

Philosophy

We adhere to a student-centered teaching and learning philosophy. We believe that students are adult learners and that each individual brings a unique set of life skills and lived experiences to the academic and practice environment. Faculty role-model and expect civility, professionalism, and active engagement from all students.

Most colleges and universities require faculty members to develop a teaching philosophy to include in their annual evaluations, dossiers for promotion and tenure, and other professional documents. If you have not developed your teaching philosophy, or you are dissatisfied with your current one, the next section provides a few suggestions to create or revise your philosophy.

Teaching Philosophy Tips and Reflections

To create your teaching philosophy, find a quiet place to reflect and contemplate without interruption. Consider the aspects of nursing education that inspire you to teach and contribute to student learning and understanding. After you consider the questions that follow shortly, share your responses with a teaching colleague to get his or her thoughts about your teaching—invite colleagues to visit your classroom to observe your teaching style, or request a classroom observation and assessment from the university's center for teaching and learning to gain further insight into your teaching.

Give some thought to the following questions:

1. What do you find enjoyable and rewarding about teaching and learning?

2. What are the basic principles and tenets that underlie your teaching?

3. What drives your passion for teaching and learning?

4. What makes you special in your role as a teacher?

5. What makes your teaching unique?

6. What pedagogical gifts do you bring to the academic environment?

7. How do others describe your teaching?

8. What aspects of teaching and learning are you really passionate about?

9. How do you establish rapport with students?

10. What do you want your students to learn?

11. How do you evaluate whether you have accomplished your teaching-learning goals?

Discovering and crafting a teaching philosophy can be a thoughtful journey and a personal capture of your deeply held beliefs about teaching and learning. Parker Palmer (1998) reminds teachers that "we teach who we are" (p. xi), meaning our approach to the classroom speaks volumes about our beliefs and values. When we reflect on and ponder our beliefs and assumptions about teaching and learning, they will reveal themselves more readily. Two abbreviated teaching philosophies are provided in the following sidebars as examples—one is from my colleague Dr. Pam Gehrke, and the other is mine. We share our philosophies with students on the first day of class.

DR. PAM GEHRKE'S PHILOSOPHY OF TEACHING AND LEARNING

My beliefs about teaching and learning emerge from the notion that the most meaningful and deep learning occurs when we engage in learning together. Each of us has much to offer as we teach one another and learn together. I assume responsibility to provide enthusiasm, respect, and excellent opportunities for learning. As teacher, I coach, mentor, facilitate, urge, prod, and question learners to develop thinking and actions based on solid evidence, rationale, and professional values. I, too, am a learner, gaining new insight from your experiences, questions, and creativity.

Learners have important responsibilities to invest in their own and each other's learning. Students in past classes have said talking and writing about course ideas with others were key to learning how political ideas apply to one's own professional nursing identity. Learners' experiences in their lives, in nursing, and as members of a profession add richness to learning, making it personal, real, and meaningful. Current issues, events, and information are catalysts for inquiry, analysis, discovery, and action as we learn together about health and policy advocacy. My goal is to empower learners to think broadly about their nursing roles, participate actively in shaping their profession, and influence conditions for health in their organizations, communities, nation, and world.

DR. CLARK'S PHILOSOPHY OF TEACHING AND LEARNING

I thoroughly enjoy teaching, interacting with students, and engaging students in the learning process. I believe that all students are experienced adult learners, capable of deep learning and of achieving substantial personal and professional goals. I believe each student brings a wealth of life, work, and educational experience to the learning environment; thus, each student adds value and meaning to the educational experience.

continues

continued

This course is designed to prepare nursing students for leadership and management roles in a variety of healthcare environments. As such, I am intentional about practical application and relevance of the material to nursing practice and to real life.

As teachers and learners in higher education, we are charged with fostering debate, challenging ideas, engaging students in intellectual inquiry, and advancing discovery. These stimulating and important discussions require all of us to bring civility to discourse and respect to our conversations and encounters. Therefore, co-creating classroom norms on the first day of class is an essential component to the leadership course. I am deeply committed to fostering a classroom environment conducive to student learning, meaningful engagement, and evocative dialogue. As a professor of higher education and as a nurse leader, I take seriously the importance of professional role-modeling as well as the intentional socialization of students into the nursing profession.

Teaching philosophies can be lengthy, but for the purposes of sharing them with students, use a shrink-wrapped approach and share an abbreviated version of your teaching philosophy. Consider publishing the abbreviated or distilled version in your course syllabus to use as a talking point. I candidly share and discuss my abbreviated philosophy with my students. To do so, I project my teaching philosophy on a large screen and ask for a student volunteer to stand and read the first two sentences aloud in class. I especially want the first sentences to strike a positive chord, so I write: "I thoroughly enjoy teaching, interacting with students, and engaging students in the learning process. I believe that all students are experienced adult learners and capable of deep learning and of achieving substantial personal and professional goals." My teaching philosophy illustrates additional key points that are important to share and discuss with my students. The second paragraph provides a solid foundation for co-creating classroom and clinical norms with my students. Because institutions of higher education are charged with engaging students in evocative dialogue and absorbing them in controversial topics and arguments, we must establish classroom norms to create a safe environment in which to argue, discuss, and allow opposing ideas to flourish.

Ken Blanchard, a leadership scholar, once said, "A river without banks is a pond." Similarly, I contend that any organization (including the classroom) devoid of norms is a rudderless ship. Thus, co-creating classroom and clinical norms is essential to successful teaching and learning and should never be underestimated. I progress from the macro to the micro to help my students understand the importance of co-creating norms. From the boardroom to the bedside, from the president's suite to the classroom, we must establish behavioral norms upon which faculty and students agree. Faculty may begin the process of co-creating classroom norms by describing the institution's vision and mission, defining civility, and discussing the university's shared values—and how each provides a foundation upon which the vision of the college and school of nursing is based. If your nursing program has developed and implemented a set of behavioral norms, share them with your students and use those as a platform to co-create classroom and clinical norms (see the following sidebar). The exemplar includes the assumption of goodwill—in other words, believing that others function from a position of respect and that uncivil behaviors are unintended. If, however, you question the intent of another, it is important to check your assumption by speaking directly to your colleague. It is essential to listen carefully and with intention, ask for what you need to resolve the matter, and hold yourself and any other(s) accountable to effectively manage the conflict.

SCHOOL OF NURSING BEHAVIORAL NORMS (EXEMPLAR)

- *Assume goodwill and best intentions*
- *Be respectful in our interactions*
- *Use direct communication (take and send the mail to the right address)*
- *Role-model professionalism, civility, and ethical conduct*
- *Listen carefully and with intention to understand*
- *Be open to other points of view*
- *Engage in respectful and constructive conflict negotiation*
- *Avoid judging and personalizing interactions*
- *Hold ourselves and each other accountable for abiding by our norms*

After explaining the value and importance of co-creating norms and discussing the example of norms in your nursing program, it's your turn to facilitate the co-creation of your classroom norms by asking, "What behaviors do you want to see in class, and what behaviors do you *not* want to see in class?" Then, determine and agree upon expected behavioral norms; ask a student volunteer to type up the norms on his or her laptop and email them to you so that you can post the norms on your online course site and paste them on an index card to distribute during the next class meeting. I requested that students bring their name tents along with a copy of their classroom norms to each class, because we would refer to them over the course of the semester.

We also co-created norms in our clinical group, and involved our community partners (preceptors) in the process so that they would have a voice in how we behaved together in our clinical groups. It is everyone's responsibility to reinforce and monitor adherence to the norms, and at midterm, we conducted a formal evaluation of how the norms were working. I am constantly amazed at how well students engaged in this process; from the very young to the more mature students, everyone valued a defined set of rules on ways to behave with one another. An example of our co-created classroom and clinical norms is provided in the following sidebar.

DR. CLARK'S CLASSROOM NORMS

- *Engage in respectful interactions*
- *Listen well while others are speaking*
- *Assume goodwill; encourage and inspire each other*
- *Respect differences and be open to other points of view*
- *Make thoughtful contributions to group work*
- *Be on time and respect one another's time*
- *Use electronic and media devices for class purposes only*
- *Sit near the door in anticipation of phone/text message*
- *HAVE FUN!*

DR. CLARK'S CLINICAL NORMS

- *Assume goodwill and best intentions*
- *Respect and celebrate differences*
- *Communicate respectfully and listen carefully*
- *Come to clinical prepared and on time*
- *Let others know right away if you need to adjust assignments or timelines*
- *Share work equally among group members*
- *Resolve conflicts directly and with respect*
- *Work hard and have fun!*

Classroom and clinical norms must be reviewed periodically, revised as needed, and reaffirmed through the course of the semester. Norms are living documents that provide a civility "touchstone" for students, faculty, and clinical partners—providing a framework for working, collaborating, and learning with and from one another. Sometimes students will suggest that they/we do not need to create "new" norms, because they have them from other classes, and they "pretty much know each other"; however, I point out that each learning environment or collection of people is unique, and, as such, we need to have our own norms. Particularly in nursing, where many of our courses are team taught, we need to be on the same page with colleagues as well as community partners in the clinical setting.

Super Threads—Course Constructs and Concepts

The most effective teachers possess a strong commitment to student learning. Bain (2004) suggests that the best teaching occurs when faculty members come to class with the intention to stimulate interest, to communicate clearly and effectively, to foster deep thinking, and to entertain multiple perspectives. Bain further explains that the best teachers use class time to help students think about information, knowledge, and ideas of the discipline. Therefore, faculty members need to cover relevant course material on the first day of class. Faculty credibility and significance of the course content are heightened by covering key concepts related to the course. Because students are often overloaded with information during the first week of classes, rather than cover highly theoretical or detailed material on the first day, I prefer to present and discuss course *super threads*—the foundational concepts that students will experience and learn about over the course of the academic term. *Super threads* are the concepts that underpin and provide a framework for a course. Think about the courses you teach, and identify the major concepts, constructs, or theoretical underpinnings that are integral to the course. Facilitate class discussion about the course super threads using pictures, famous quotes, or passages to bring the concepts alive and to strengthen students' memory and application. To correspond with the concepts of civility, professionalism, and ethical practice to ensure patient safety introduced earlier in this chapter, I have provided examples of these super threads in Figure 9.3.

CIVILITY

When we are on the receiving end of an act of civility, we feel validated, valued, and it gives our life meaning. —P. M. Forni

PROFESSIONALISM

Professional is not a label you give yourself –it's a description you hope others will apply to you. —David Maister

ETHICAL PRACTICE

It is curious that physical courage should be so common in the world, and moral courage so rare. —Mark Twain

PATIENT SAFETY

To err is human, to cover up is unforgivable, and to fail to learn is inexcusable. —Sir Liam Donaldson

FIGURE 9.3

Examples of leadership course super threads.

Finishing Touches

Nursing faculty members are encouraged to foster debate and engage students in intellectual inquiry. These activities require bringing civility to discourse and respect to our conversations and encounters. Fostering a classroom environment conducive to student learning and evocative dialogue is critical to the profession. On the first day of classes, faculty members are encouraged to devote as much time as necessary to review the syllabus, their teaching philosophy, the course goals and expectations, and the role of civil discourse. A careful review of the syllabus can be helpful in clarifying assignments, course expectations, and expected behaviors. Co-creating classroom and clinical behavioral norms forms the foundation for expected behavior in the academic and practice arena.

CIVILITY TIP

Reflect on the most important constructs and concepts contained in the classes you teach. Pick one of the courses you teach most, and consider the super threads that are foundational to the course. In other words, if your students learn little else, what do you want them to learn in the course you selected? List and describe the super threads and discuss their importance and relevance in your next scheduled class. Have some fun with the super threads, and find creative ways to integrate them into your class discussion.

Chapter 10
Scholarly Teaching, Engaged Learning, and Finding Our Joy

The mediocre teacher tells. The good teacher explains. The superior teacher demonstrates. The great teacher inspires. –William Arthur Ward

This chapter discusses:

- Defining scholarly teaching and learning
- Classroom assessment techniques
- Applying active learning strategies
- Becoming a master teacher

The Scholarship of Teaching and Learning

I have long embraced the work of Ernest Boyer (1990), who challenged faculty and academic leaders in higher education to break out of the tired old teaching-versus-research debate and define, in more creative ways, what it means to be a scholar. Boyer called for a broader definition of *scholarship* that brings legitimacy to the full scope of academic work.

Boyer wrote:

> Surely, scholarship means engaging in original research. But the work of the scholar also means stepping back from one's investigation, looking for connections, building bridges between theory and practice, and communicating one's knowledge effectively to students. Specifically, we conclude that the work of the professoriate might be thought of as having four separate, yet overlapping, functions. These are: the scholarship of discovery; the scholarship of integration; the scholarship of application; and the scholarship of teaching. (1990, p. 16)

Specifically, the scholarship of teaching includes not only transmitting knowledge, but also transforming and extending it. The scholarship of teaching was further elucidated by Lee Shulman (2011), president emeritus of the Carnegie Foundation for the Advancement of Teaching, who provided a more precise definition of the scholarship of teaching, stating that *scholarly teaching* must meet three criteria:

- The work must be made public.

- The work must be subject to peer review and evaluation.

- The work must be accessible for exchange and use by members of one's disciplinary community.

Shulman writes, "The scholarship of teaching is not synonymous with excellent teaching. It requires faculty to frame and systematically investigate questions related to student learning" (Hutchings & Shulman, 1999, p. 13). Shulman further noted that faculty must understand the discipline, the theories, and the methods of educational research to be engaged in the scholarship of teaching and learning.

So in light of this definition of scholarly teaching, what then is evidence-based teaching and learning? According to Brookfield (1995), scholarly teachers reflect on their teaching, utilize classroom assessment techniques, discuss teaching issues with colleagues, read and apply the literature of teaching and learning, and disseminate their scholarly works. Brookfield (1995, 2006) describes "good teaching" as whatever we do to help students learn and "best teaching" as critical reflection and constant scrutiny about teaching and the conditions that foster learning.

Brookfield also noted that the most important knowledge teachers need is to understand how students learn.

Teachers have at their disposal several different tools for measuring learning styles. One of my favorites is the VARK (Fleming, 2012):

- **V** stands for visual learning (learning by seeing).

- **A** stands for aural learning (learning by hearing).

- **R** stands for reading (learning by reading and writing).

- **K** stands for kinesthetic (learning by touching, holding, or feeling).

We need to understand and appreciate our students' different learning styles—and our own learning style as teachers, because we often teach in our own comfort zone. Many of our students learn differently than we do and differently than other students, so no one teaching method can effectively reach all students. Hence, we cannot employ, nor can we address, all learning styles all of the time.

Benner, Sutphen, Leonard, and Day (2010) remind us that redesigning nursing education is an urgent societal agenda and that radical changes are needed. Further, the profound changes in nursing practice call for equally profound changes in the education of nurses and the preparation of nurse educators. Similarly, the Institute of Medicine (IOM) report *The Future of Nursing: Leading Change, Advancing Health* (2011) also noted that many nursing schools have dealt with the rapid growth of health research and knowledge by compressing vast information into the curriculum and adding layers of content that require more instruction. The authors of this report called for new approaches and educational models to respond to burgeoning information in the health field. The report further urges nurses to be engaged in lifelong learning; to participate in continuing professional development; and to perform with cutting-edge competence in practice, teaching, and research. Thus, nurse educators must be prepared to promote student learning in multiple and myriad ways.

One of my favorite articles on teaching in nursing was written by Pamela Ironside and Terry Valiga in 2006. These seasoned and experienced nurse educators—and leaders in the science of teaching and learning in nursing—encourage nursing faculty to be open and responsive to students' learning needs and interests rather than being rigid, lockstep, and unyielding. Faculty need to be flexible, teach the courses about which they are passionate, and create and encourage a lively exchange of ideas. Students and teachers must openly discuss significant and controversial issues, embrace diverse thinking, and explore conflicting views and perspectives (Ironside & Valiga, 2006). I believe that when faculty heed this constructive advice, we are better positioned to prevent classroom disruption and disturbance.

The more we engage students in active learning activities, the less likely the potential for uncivil and disruptive behavior. Involving students in active learning strategies minimizes disruption by promoting cooperation and collaboration (Clark, 2009). Using active learning strategies and team activities helps students stay focused and motivated. Making learning meaningful and applicable by using stories, real-life examples, case-based scenarios, and group discussion minimizes incivility. Because significant learning takes place outside the classroom, faculty can encourage students to practice and apply what they have learned in class to their lives outside the classroom. These strategies and interventions help to create safe, civil teaching-learning environments (Clark & Davis-Kenaley, 2011).

Beginning With the End in Mind

I would like to share an experience I had several years ago with the director of the Center for Teaching and Learning at Boise State University. Dr. Susan Shadle is a gifted chemistry professor, brilliant scholar, keen observer—and my cherished friend. For years, I taught a multidisciplinary, elective Adolescent Mental Health course. The course was available to students from all majors across campus. I thoroughly enjoyed teaching the course and spent numerous hours developing it, making it the best course possible by asking students for continuous feedback to improve the content and course delivery. I met with Susan to get her expert opinion on the course. I was very pleased with it, students were thriving, and I was certain that Susan would be impressed and give it her seal of approval.

Prior to our meeting, Susan reviewed my course syllabus, textbook, and class assignments. My hope was for Susan to provide suggestions to tweak the course and make some slight improvements, so I was completely unprepared for what she had to say. Susan gazed at me with her intelligent eyes and asked, "Cindy, what is your primary objective— the number one outcome you want your students to learn by taking this course? If your students learn only one thing, what do you want it to be?" I looked at her thoughtfully, but I had no immediate reply. It slowly occurred to me that I had not developed the course and its assignments with the "end in mind." In fact, I had to deliberate for several long minutes to finally respond to Susan's question.

Finally, I said, "By the end of the term, I want each student to appreciate the adolescent experience, to view adolescents as a special population, and to dispel the myriad stereotypes that surround this group."

Susan looked at me and said, "That's great; however, your syllabus and course assignments are not constructed to reach this goal."

I was flabbergasted. I was silent for a moment and then responded, "You're right." Susan and I spent the next 2 hours discussing the importance of student learning. It was an exhilarating discovery for me. After our meeting, there was no turning back. I knew that each course, each class, and each objective must be carefully considered in relationship to student learning.

Teaching without learning is just talking. (Angelo & Cross, 1993)

What Are CATs?

Beginning on the day I met with Susan, I began incorporating Classroom Assessment Techniques (CATs) into all of my classes to be sure I was meeting the intended course and class objectives. More specifically, I used CATs to assess learning outcomes and to help frame what I wanted my students to learn. Too often we assume that students are learning what we are trying to teach them, yet when we begin to grade exams and assignments, we might realize that students are not learning as well as we expected. We might clearly see a gap between what is being taught and what is being learned. If we are relying exclusively on summative course evaluations, we might notice these gaps in learning too late and be unable to remedy the problem. Using CATs can promote student learning, improve the effectiveness of our teaching, and allow both teachers and students to improve the quality of learning (Angelo & Cross, 1993). Though we need to use both formative and summative evaluations to improve teaching and learning, we must also use frequent formative assessments (e.g., CATs) to evaluate students' understanding of course content. Formative evaluations also allow for the evaluation of teaching strategies and student learning outcomes in a fluid and dynamic manner.

Many faculty have expressed serious concern about higher education's heavy reliance on summative student evaluations of faculty and course instruction to inform decisions about faculty promotion and tenure, advancement, and compensation. To some extent, I share their concern, and highly recommend the use of ongoing formative evaluations throughout the course term. When faculty rely on summative student evaluations, they run the risk of a low percentage of students completing them, of students with an ax to grind being the ones to respond, or of questions on the evaluation being poorly framed to address the ways in which students learn. In any case, faculty should collect ongoing, formative evaluative data to augment or complement summative evaluations. Faculty need to quantify the evaluative data, summarize the findings in retrievable documents, and place them in personal files that are easy to access when needed.

I like to implement one of my favorite CATs at midterm of the semester. The midterm CAT is completely anonymous; I do not ask for names so that the students can be as candid as possible. Students respond to the questions in the following list (the fifth question being optional). The questions are carefully framed to gather information about instruction and student learning. Because I am also interested in assessing the effectiveness of our classroom norms, I include a question about them. Midterm CAT questions are:

1. What about this course and its instruction foster your learning?

2. What about this course and its instruction present a barrier to your learning?

3. In your opinion, how are our classroom norms working? And what suggestions do you have to improve their effectiveness?

4. What suggestions do you have to improve your learning in this course?

5. On average, how many hours each week do you spend engaged in activities that bring you joy? What brings you joy?

After the students complete the midterm CAT, I conduct a qualitative analysis of their responses, quantify and post the themes online, provide a summarized hard copy—and most importantly, I engage the students in conversation during the next class meeting. We discuss the CAT results and identify specific strategies to improve the quality and delivery of the course. The fifth question is always interesting and elicits lively conversation between and among my students and me because we place a high premium on stress management, self-care, and finding joy beyond the classroom and the workplace.

I am also a big fan of "1-minute free writes"—an assessment that students can complete quickly using 3x5-inch index cards. If you are curious about whether the class topic was understood by your students, you can assess their learning by asking them to use one side of the 3x5 index card to identify the most significant point or concept they learned today and then to flip the card and identify the one point or concept they need to learn more about. I literally give my students 1 minute to complete the exercise. The goal is to elicit their most salient thoughts—and use as little class time as possible. The 3x5 index cards are perfect for this exercise because they gather brief, pithy, relevant responses from students. I collect this information anonymously to obtain the most honest responses possible from my students and then use the results to guide my course preparation for the next class or clinical period.

You might want to design your own method for assessment. I also use this 3x5 index card technique to periodically evaluate our classroom norms. On the front side of the card, I ask students to evaluate the effectiveness of our norms and then flip the card over and make suggestions as to how our norms might be improved. After class, I conduct an analysis to identify and quantify themes, post them on my course site, and discuss the findings with students during our next class. This technique can also be used to evaluate the effectiveness of the norms that have been created in the clinical setting with students, faculty, and community partners.

Assessing Student Self-Perceptions of Civility

In Chapter 5, I mentioned one of my favorite exercises designed to assess students' self-perception of their level of civility (and incivility) as adult learners. The Clark Civility Index for Students is an evidence-based tool that can be completed individually by students at any time—though it's preferable to have students complete the index early in the term or during new-student orientation. The index can also be used to assess their classmates' perceived level of civility and incivility once students have gotten to know one another as a cohort and have enough experience as classmates to effectively evaluate them. In either case, the purpose of the activity is to raise awareness, generate discussion, discuss varying perceptions of civility and incivility, and develop ways to improve civility acumen.

When orienting new nursing students to the program, I have them complete the Civility Index for Students based on their perceptions of themselves. Students complete the index anonymously. I do not ask for any identifying information because this elimination encourages students to provide honest, candid responses. After completing the index, I facilitate discussion based on student feedback related to the items. For example, item #11 asks students for their opinion as to how often they address disruptive student behaviors and promote a safe, civil learning environment. Actually, there is no right or wrong response. Instead, I am more interested in the discussion that follows.

For example, in one of my classes, we had a rousing discussion as to whether or not the disruptive behavior should be addressed each time it occurs or only if it is a pattern of behavior, and if it is addressed, how might this happen in a respectful manner. This is amazing subject matter to immerse students in a deeper discussion of fostering civility. After our discussion, I collect the indices and collate student responses so that I can present the aggregated results during the next class. This collection of rich information is fodder for continued discussion.

At other times, I have used the index to gather student perceptions of both self and classmates. Once the students get to know each other, I distribute the index with a copy printed on each side of the paper—on the front side of the paper, I ask the students to respond to the index questions by asking "How often do I…?" and on the other side of the paper, I ask the students to think about their classmates and respond to each item asking, "How often do my classmates—?" This exercise is an interesting one because in nearly every case, students rate themselves higher on every item than they rate their classmates. Once again, the conversation this activity generates is impressive. Similar to the individualized exercise, I do not ask for identifying information. After class, I collate the responses to show comparisons between self and others during the next class. The discussion that ensues is generally spirited and thought-provoking. The index is provided in Chapter 5.

Active Learning Strategies for the Classroom

Involving students in active learning strategies minimizes classroom incivility and disruption by promoting cooperation, collaboration, and mutual goal setting (Clark, 2009; Gonzalez & Lopez, 2001; Nilson, 2003). Active learning strategies also increase student participation and teamwork (Billings & Halstead, 2016), enhance student achievement and productivity, promote positive interpersonal relationships, and foster psychological health (Nilson, 2003). Designing and implementing active learning strategies require a paradigm shift for both students and faculty. Students must move from a more passive listening and note-taking role to a more active problem-solving and discovery role. Students must also learn to work in teams and communities, to collaborate with peers, and to view faculty as facilitators of learning rather than simply as imparters of knowledge and information.

The faculty role must change as well. The primary goal is to shift from being the "expert" to becoming the facilitator of student learning and engagement. For some faculty, making this adjustment can be difficult and uncomfortable. The faculty role in an active learning environment is to guide students to function effectively as members of a team and to empower each team member to feel a sense of personal responsibility for the success of his or her teammates. In other words, team members must feel they need one another to accomplish an achievable and relevant goal. Therefore, faculty need to be very clear about the activity's purpose, goal(s), and rationale for using the technique. The students should be given specific outcomes and timelines for completion.

As nursing faculty, we can draw from our physician colleagues such as Stanford School of Medicine (2016) to further understand educational transformation in the health sciences. Like nursing, medical education is shifting to the pedagogy of interactive learning, which engages the learner to interact with the course material. It reinvigorates the classroom for both students and faculty by converting lectures into discussions and provides opportunities for problem-solving and applied learning. One example is the "flipped classroom" where students come to class with sufficient background information and content understanding to participate in higher-level discussions and to engage with the material in a meaningful way.

Some of the benefits of interactive learning include enhanced understanding, retention, and motivation; a deepened exploration of the course material through real-world applications; and the opportunity to make meaningful connections between what they are learning and its relevance to clinical practice. Interactive learning also involves an avenue for giving and receiving immediate feedback, opportunities for close interaction with faculty and peers, and a venue for collaborative construction of knowledge and clinical application. When "real life" clinical scenarios are simulated and de-briefed, learners are more likely to "think like a nurse."

When learning begins prior to class through the use of anticipatory activities, online videos, just-in-time teaching (JiTT), and similar strategies, class time is freed up for experiential learning. A shift to active learning strategies provides a rich forum for student and faculty interaction and making real-world applications through problem-solving, case studies, team-based learning, and other group activities. The immense (and continuously growing) volume of nursing knowledge and increasing complexity of the healthcare environment require new educational pedagogies and technologies. Today's team-based healthcare requires the ability to work closely with individuals from diverse backgrounds to solve patient problems that are too complex to be solved by one discipline or individual (Stanford School of Medicine, 2016).

I highly encourage nurse educators to implement active learning strategies in their nursing courses and throughout the program curriculum. By doing so they can gain several advantages including cultivating a deeper interest in learning, increased critical-thinking and problem-solving skills, and an enhanced level of teamwork (Billings & Halstead, 2016). A well-structured learning activity fosters learner independence and creativity while working to achieve the course outcomes. As I noted earlier, nurse educators need to assess active learning activities on a continuous basis; these ongoing formative evaluations appraise learning activities throughout the course, assess student learning, and help to identify strategies to improve the quality of the learning experience.

In the next section, I have provided several teaching-learning strategies that faculty can use to minimize academic incivility, foster faculty-student relationships, and enhance student engagement and learning. However, please remember, all suggested active learning strategies to promote civility and engagement are contextual and situated within the individual academic culture and nursing program. They are also largely reliant upon each educator's unique teaching philosophy, style, technique, and delivery methods.

Think, Pair, Square, Share Activity

The think, pair, square, share activity can be used with small or large classroom sizes and is a great way to generate discussion, critical thinking, and theory-to-practice application. To get started, consider a provocative and engaging question or problem. You might also begin with a planned question or problem to open the dialogue on a given topic, and then continue by asking succeeding questions based on student responses. This type of spontaneous questioning is referred to as the Socratic method. If you are uncomfortable with this method, you can use a more structured activity to generate discussion. For example, if the course topic is on healthcare finance and fiscal management, you might pose the following question: "Based on your readings for today's class and your experiences in the clinical setting, how might nurses be effective stewards of limited financial and human resources in the healthcare environment?" Or if you are teaching a pharmacology course on the use of psychotropic medications with the elderly, you might pose the following problem: "According to a recent meta-analysis, elderly patients who take psychotropic drugs have an increased risk of falling. As members of the nurse-led committee assigned to prevent and reduce falls in your long-term facility, what recommendations will you make to protect the patients?"

After the question or problem is posed, have students first think quietly about their response or solution to the problem and then have them pair up with another student sitting near them to share their thoughts and suggestions, then one pair of students will join (square up) with another pair of students to further discuss the issue. This iteration creates a synergy and an expansion of critical thinking and thoughtful application to situations well beyond the ideas generated by a single individual. Have a member of each group report to the larger group to continue discussion and problem-solving on a larger scale.

Free Writes

Free writes are an excellent way to cultivate thinking and construct ideas. Grammar, spelling, and punctuation do not matter. The goal is to get as many thoughts as possible down on paper (or by using a keyboard) about a specific topic within a 2- to 3-minute time frame. Free writes serve as effective warm-up exercises for class discussion and help get the cognitive juices flowing. Many times students come to class having forgotten the topic discussed in previous class sessions or the focus of the class readings. To get their "heads in the game," you might write three key points on the board and have the students free write for 1 minute on each key point. For example, if the class topic is fluids and electrolytes, you might include the following key points:

1. Requirements for electrolyte balance

2. Renal regulation

3. Fluid movement

You might also construct a class free write using a "seed sentence" such as, "Important principles of fluid, electrolyte, and nutrition management include _____ [fill in the blank]." Then have students write their reactions to the statement.

Free writes can also be assigned as homework. To increase student reading and comprehension, have students write three summarizing statements after reading each major section or chapter of the assignment. As a rule, these are not formally graded; instead, you can collect them as evidence that students have completed the reading and free write assignment. You can count free writes as part of class participation or as "ungraded but required" assignments.

Anticipatory Activities

Anticipatory activities are reflective homework assignments completed by students outside of the classroom that set the stage for active class discussion and participation. Students are assigned course readings and then asked to respond to thought-provoking questions that prepare them to participate in an in-class exercise that reveals their knowledge acquisition and learning of the content material.

Developing anticipatory activities is an excellent way for faculty to express their creativity and pedagogical aptitude. Think about what makes your teaching special or exceptional and then incorporate these methods into the student assignment. I love storytelling and narrative pedagogy. So, in my anticipatory assignments, I often ask students to include a personal story about the course topic. For example, if the day's topic centers around ethical decision-making, after students complete the course readings, I give the following assignment:

1. In advance of class, consider various ethical dilemmas that might occur with the patient population at your current clinical site. Please discuss with your preceptor (or community partner) real or possible ethical dilemmas that might occur among the population of patients you are working with this semester.

2. After you've identified a possible ethical dilemma, write a brief summary of the ethical dilemma, how it impacted you, and how you resolved it (or did not resolve it).

3. Bring your ethical dilemma(s) and written summary to class.

4. Students will break into groups, discuss each student's ethical dilemma examples, select one dilemma, and use all the elements of an ethical decision-making model to resolve it.

Some of the ethical dilemmas that students have recently shared include being assigned to care for a patient (prisoner) convicted of child rape and other crimes against children and caring for an HIV-positive patient who has not disclosed their illness to the health department.

After the students have identified and processed an ethical dilemma using an evidence-based decision model, they synthesize their group discussion into a single "gem" or "pearl" to share with the class. The "gem" or "pearl" might be a provocative question for discussion, a key concept or discovery, or an interesting idea to engage the class in discussion. This synthesis is an important aspect of learning. A synthesis is not a summary; instead it is an opportunity to create new knowledge out of existing knowledge, and to use this new information to develop a cogent argument or a unique perspective on a broader topic.

Just-in-Time Teaching (JiTT)

Just-in-time teaching (JiTT) is another active learning strategy designed to engage students in learning new material by responding to questions ahead of or during class to provide the faculty with information about students' knowledge prior to class. With JiTT, students answer and submit a set of questions before class begins based on the learning objectives related to upcoming course material. JiTT questions should be relatively brief and take students about 15 to 30 minutes to complete. You may wish to include questions asking what is most important, interesting, or confusing about the material. Once submitted, the faculty reviews the student responses and develops in-class learning activities to address learning gaps and to build on existing knowledge. Here are some sample questions:

1. Briefly summarize your understanding of the class material.

2. What aspects of the material are you unclear or uncertain about?

3. What aspects of the material require a deeper discussion and application during class?

It is important to maintain a firm link between the JiTT questions and in-class activities. Student responses can be used to craft active learning experiences such as small-group exercises based on representative samples from the full set of responses. Using verbatim responses often makes class more interesting and student focused. The use of Socratic questioning can help bring the material and discussion alive. A Socratic approach to teaching is one in which faculty pose thoughtful questions to help students think, reflect, and learn. This approach helps students construct knowledge, hone problem-solving skills, and improve long-term retention of knowledge (Science Education Resource Center at Carleton College, 2016). The nearby sidebar includes tips for teachers and examples of utilizing Socratic questioning.

TIPS FOR TEACHERS

- *Plan significant questions that provide structure and direction to the lesson.*

- *Phrase the questions clearly and specifically.*

- *Wait Time: Maintain silence and wait at least 5 to 15 seconds (or for as much time as needed) for students to respond.*

- *Keep the discussion focused.*

- *Follow up on students' responses and invite elaboration.*

- *Stimulate the discussion with probing questions.*

- *Periodically summarize (or have students summarize) what has been discussed.*

- *Draw as many students as possible into the discussion.*

- *Do not pose yes/no questions, as they do little to promote thinking or encourage discussion.*

- *Do not pose questions that are vague, ambiguous, or beyond the level of the students.*

Source: http://serc.carleton.edu/sp/library/socratic/fourth.html (How to Use the Socratic Method in the Classroom, n.d.)

Here are some examples for Socratic questioning.

- *Could you elaborate further?*

- *Can you give us an example?*

continues

continued

- *How might you verify or test that assumption?*

- *Could you be more specific by providing some examples?*

- *What are some of the challenges for the healthcare team regarding the complexity of this patient condition?*

- *How might we look at this in other ways?*

- *What might other members of the healthcare team (including the patient and his/her family) think about your approach?*

- *Is this the most important problem or issue to consider for this patient?*

Case Studies

Case studies can be useful teaching tools; they help students learn how to solve open-ended, high uncertainty problems that have more than one workable solution, though some might be better than others (Nilson, 2003). Case studies expose students to real-world situations and challenge them to apply course knowledge to analyze issues and solve problems. Many textbooks include examples of case studies; however, you can write your own to suit your instructional purposes. Doing so will get your storytelling and creative juices flowing. Teachers typically enjoy case studies because they require students to be actively engaged in the application of the course content, assist in problem-solving, foster high-level critical thinking skills, and increase student involvement.

Faculty can use a case study with the entire class or use a small-group discussion format. I prefer a combination of both by having small-group discussions that build to include the entire class. Continuing with the example of my class on ethical decision-making, all groups work on the same case study with the proviso that each group reaches a consensus on its answers and is prepared to summarize them for the class (see the case study depicted in the accompanying sidebar). Students assemble in groups, consider the case study, apply this dilemma to an ethical decision-making model, and report the "gems" and "pearls" of their group discussion. The general class discussion helps to create an inspired level of large-group dialogue.

THE CASE OF THE PHARMACEUTICAL COMPANY—EXEMPLAR

You are the director of clinical services at a large medical center. Your position places you in contact with many pharmaceutical company representatives. Recently, you were offered an opportunity to fly to San Francisco for a week (all expenses paid by the pharmaceutical company) to attend a conference on a revolutionary new cardiac medication developed by their company. Your medical center is the leading cardiac center in the state. No explicit mention of expected reciprocation has been stated. Using the MORAL model of ethical decision-making, how will you decide what to do?

I would like to illustrate another case study example I have used to expose students to real-world situations and challenge them to apply course knowledge to analyze and solve problems. The learning objectives include:

1. Function as a member of an Ethics Team in healthcare to review and resolve an ethical dilemma (ED)

2. Apply an evidence-based Ethical Decision Making Tool to resolve the dilemma

3. Analyze the efficacy of the resolution of the ED in small and large groups

Prior to class, students are randomly assigned to act as members of an Ethics Team. Roles include a charge nurse, social worker, chaplain, physician, nurse ethicist, and a community member. A week before class begins, each student is expected to examine the perspective of the role to which she or he is assigned. For example, if a student is assigned the role of the chaplain, he or she needs to learn about the role in order to express this perspective as a member of the Ethics Team. The number of Ethics Teams depends on class size. Because my classes generally consisted of 75 students, I had approximately 12 teams.

After assembling into their teams and reviewing and discussing the Case of Theo (see nearby sidebar), students collaborate to resolve the dilemma from the point of view of the role they were assigned. In other words, the student playing the role of the nurse responded from the viewpoint of a nurse, the student playing the role of the chaplain responded from the perspective of a chaplain, and so forth. This allows nursing students to consider and value other points of view and to improve communication among members of the healthcare team. After the students have processed and resolved the ethical dilemma, a spokesperson for each Ethics Team presents their findings and rationale to the large group as if the group is the patient/family.

THE CASE OF THEO—EXEMPLAR

Several years ago, a 17-year-old adolescent (Theo) needed a liver transplant. He was a high school dropout, was living with a girlfriend who was 2 months pregnant by him and already had a 2-year-old child. Theo's liver disease was related to chronic methamphetamine and alcohol abuse. His stepfather was eligible for Medicaid, and Theo was accepted for (and given) a new liver.

After the transplant, Theo abided by the immunosuppressive drug regimen while he was under medical and nursing staff care. However, once discharged, he did not follow his care plan and took his immunosuppressive drugs sporadically. Theo was incarcerated for assault and battery on his girlfriend and returned to using drugs and alcohol. His liver began to fail. He returned to the medical clinic where the medical team determined that he needed another liver transplant. You are a member of the Ethics Team charged with making a decision about Theo's need for a liver transplant—using the 4-Boxes Ethical Decision Making Tool (Jonsen, Siegler, & Winslade, 2010), what will the team decide?

Though case studies/scenarios have been used in nursing for many years, unfolding case studies are gaining attention. Unfolding case studies tell a continuous story in segments over real or condensed time. Because real-life situations usually evolve and change over time, this structure adds realism. Lisa Day (2011) has written an excellent paper about how nurse educators can transform lecture notes into an unfolding case study. The unfolding narrative (patient's story) provides an engaged learning experience to draw out students' concerns and questions. Rather than presenting several text-laden slides, the unfolding case study engages students in dialogue about delivering the best care that nurses need to provide in a particular situation. As the case studies unfold, lectures will have a small, or nonexistent, role. By centering class discussion on the unfolding case study, students and their teacher engage in creative problem-solving together.

Structured Academic Controversy

Structured Academic Controversy (SAC) is an active learning strategy in which students learn about and discuss a controversial issue from multiple perspectives. SAC engages students in argument, encourages them to apply decision-making and problem-solving skills, and guides them to seek consensus using a culminating question. Unlike conventional debates that result in a "winner," SAC encourages students to consider multiple solutions to controversial issues and produce varying perspectives and solutions. The SAC format depends on your class time frame, learning objectives, and instructional goals—and can be used to address vexing issues that arouse sensitivities. During the 2012 election season, I facilitated class using SAC to address the topic of healthcare reform. I had my students prepare for class by reading general background information on the issue. Then, I had them browse the presidential candidates' official websites and peruse other readings regarding each candidate's position and political platform on healthcare reform. Students also prepared three to four questions they would like to ask the candidate on the topic of healthcare reform.

On the class day when the topic of healthcare reform was discussed, I met the students at the door and asked them to pick a card on which I had printed the presidential candidate's name. I gave out eight cards total. Four of the cards included the name of the Republican candidate, and the other four cards included the name of the Democratic candidate. The students representing each candidate were assigned to debate the healthcare reform issues. The students not assigned a card (political party) became part of the "town hall" audience and directed specific healthcare-reform questions to classmates representing members of each political party. Because of the potential for heated and spirited debate (and maybe even incivility), I reviewed classroom norms with students before engaging in the SAC experience. For example, I emphasized certain norms such as speaking one at a time, listening well, and responding respectfully, and using reasoned and measured discourse.

To begin the SAC debate, each political side presented their position on healthcare reform. Next, members of the town hall audience asked questions about healthcare reform to each political group. The role of faculty is to monitor the "debate" and to keep the discussion civil. After the town hall audience was finished asking questions, the faculty posed a "culminating question" that refocused the discussion. In this case, the culminating question that I asked students was this: "Based on what we know about the current state of healthcare reform and what we have learned today, what is the role of nursing in advancing healthcare reform in the United States?" This culminating question was designed to engage students in discussing the role of nursing, rather than focusing on who "won" the debate or on which political position is best.

This particular teaching strategy affords students an explicit opportunity to express their personal opinions about the controversial topic of presidential politics. This experience allows students from each side of the ideological and political spectrum, those who believe vehemently in their own political ideals, to practice and demonstrate civility while continuing to argue passionately for their individual beliefs. My goal was to facilitate a free, vigorous, and respectful pursuit of ideas—this strikes at the very core of higher education.

My experience with SAC has been extraordinary. I often end the class with a "One-Minute CAT"—I ask on one side of a 3x5 index card, "What do you know now that you didn't know last week?" and on the other side of the 3x5 index card, "How will you use this knowledge in your nursing practice?" I am constantly amazed at the high level of student engagement and learning in this type of activity. I highly recommend it to faculty, but only after careful preparation and only strategically placed in the academic term when classroom norms are functional and well-established.

Student Quote of the Week

I am so impressed with my colleague's approach to increasing student involvement in our school of nursing's writing intensive course. Dr. Pam Gehrke teaches a required senior level nursing course titled "Policy, Power & Voice." In this course, students' written and oral voices aid them in learning political concepts, discussing ideas with one another, and practicing the use of political concepts in nursing situations. One of Pam's learning objectives is to give students an expanded and changed view of nursing (Gehrke, 2012); she does this by using specific and intentional teaching strategies to promote such change. One of her strategies includes the "Quote of the Week." In this assignment, students answer weekly homework questions. Those are turned in, read, and graded by Pam, and returned to students with feedback. Students' written work frequently leads Pam to re-examine ideas, gain new insights, and find inspiration in their expressions and voices.

As a way of promoting the shared wisdom nurses hold as colleagues, she posts a "Quote of the Week" on the course site at the conclusion of each class week by choosing an insightful, stimulating quote from a student. In the live classroom, Pam starts each new class by showing and reading these quotes, giving the prominence of place by emphasizing students' voices and linking their ideas to the new topic for each week. In the online class, students receive the "Quote of the Week" via email, making it more likely to be seen and read. On the first day of class, Pam tells students she will be doing this and gives them the opportunity to opt out with no penalty. She is selective and judicious in choosing quotes, avoiding anything that might seem too personal or potentially embarrassing. The "Quote of the Week" has provided opportunities to feature many "quiet voices" in classes whose oral voices might not always be heard. Students' responses have been enthusiastic, and the "Quote of the Week" placed onscreen instantly quiets the classroom, as students seem to enjoy seeing what their classmates have said. Two examples of student "Quotes of the Week" include:

> Compliments are like seeds that can blossom into something unexpectedly wonderful. Now, I seem to find myself learning something new about my chosen profession every day we talk.

> We are nurses-to-be, but we could be the generation that changes the image of nursing and bolsters nursing power.

Change-the-Date Option

My friend and colleague Dr. Susan Luparell is a masterful and gifted teacher who has a wealth of experience with incorporating teaching tips into her classes. These teaching tips show deep respect for the adult learners, help to reduce incivility, and, most importantly, engage them in the learning process. Susan offers the following teaching tip that has made a particular difference in her classes. It's called the "Change-the-Date Option."

CHANGE-THE-DATE OPTION
DR. SUSAN LUPARELL

I draw heavily on adult learning theory in my teaching practice, and I find the Change-the-Date Option to be highly consistent with this theory. We know as faculty that our students, perhaps now more than ever, have many competing responsibilities and demands on their time. It is not at all uncommon these days for a full-time student to be working more than 20 hours per week and also managing a family. Unfortunately, the traditional approach to nursing education is not often able to take this into account, and we generally schedule overall courses and specific assignments in a manner that focuses more on faculty needs or a rather arbitrary time frame. Even if we tried to be highly responsive to students' responsibilities in our scheduling of due dates, it would be virtually impossible to meet the individual needs of an entire classroom of students. The Change-the-Date Option gives the student a say in when an assignment will be due and, I think, demonstrates value and respect for their time and other responsibilities.

It works like this: For any one assignment during the semester (other than exams), the student may opt to change the due date to a time more suitable for them. I require no explanation or justification at all and the student may choose to exercise the option at any point up to the minute the assignment is due. All they need to do is notify me that they will be exercising the option. We then negotiate a new due date that is mutually

> *agreeable, although I do retain the final say because of semester or other important deadlines. For team-based assignments, the entire team must collectively exercise the option.*
>
> *Students have exercised the option for any number of reasons over the years—for example, when they need more time to do a good job on the assignment at hand in my class, when they need additional time to focus on an assignment in another class, or when a last-minute opportunity to do something fun with friends or family has arisen and would otherwise not be possible. However, my experience has shown that students are very judicious in their use of the Change-the-Date Option, and most never use it. Nonetheless, they seem to really appreciate its availability, and I believe it pays dividends in establishing a trusting classroom where students feel valued.*

This Change-the-Date Option affords students the opportunity to take charge of their own learning. When pressure builds and the potential for incivility increases, students can negotiate an assignment deadline to spend time with loved ones or to improve their assignment; this puts the student in charge and diffuses a possible conflicted or stressful outcome. When faculty and students collaborate and when faculty treat students with respect and consideration, it is a win-win situation. When students and faculty share a mutual respect and enjoy a positive teacher-student relationship, the benefits are many. Students are more likely to be interested in the course content, demonstrate higher levels of academic achievement, and cause fewer classroom disruptions.

Using Standardized Participants (SPs) to Address Nurse Incivility: An Exemplar

Unfortunately, new graduate nurses are experiencing incivility both in the practice setting and in some cases the academic environment, which can result in a negative impact on their physical and mental health and well-being—and might even lead them to leave the profession altogether. Given the serious impact of incivility, nursing faculty must prepare students to identify and effectively address incivility in the practice setting (Clark & Ahten, 2011a).

> Incivility should be a concern for nurses across the spectrum of the profession, from students to educators to clinicians to managers to organizational administrators. Uncivil behaviors affect recruitment and retention in the profession. Students leave nursing programs, nurses leave the bedside, educators leave the classroom, and the profession suffers. Ultimately, the public suffers too. (Clark & Ahten, 2011a, sec. 5)

Further, the Center for American Nurses (2008), in its policy statement on lateral violence and bullying, addressed the "reality shock" experienced by new graduates being socialized into the workplace and made several recommendations for eliminating disruptive behavior in healthcare settings (Center for American Nurses, 2008, p. 6):

- Disseminate information to nurses and students that addresses conflict and provides information about how to change disruptive behavior in the workplace.

- Develop educational programs regarding bullying and strategies on how to recognize and address such disruptive behavior.

- Develop and implement curricula that educate nursing students on the incidence of disruptive behaviors including lateral violence and bullying, along with steps to take to eradicate this behavior.

Unfortunately, you find very few examples regarding the inclusion of incivility-related learning experiences into a nursing curriculum. However, you can draw similarities from Griffin (2004) and Griffin and Clark (2014), who used didactic and interactive instruction and cueing cards in an educational module on lateral violence with newly licensed nurses. Curtis, Bowen, and Reid (2007) also suggest incorporating lateral-violence awareness and associated content into nursing curricula using educational interventions focused on the identification of horizontal violence indicators, development of personal action plans for dealing with incivility in preparation for entry to practice, and opportunities for debriefing following clinical experiences. The authors strongly recommended the use of role-play as a tool for teaching assertiveness training and effective communication to minimize interpersonal conflict. Further, Curtis et al.

(2007) stressed that teaching this content and associated skills is part of the nurse educator's role.

The use of high-fidelity simulation is expanding and gaining popularity in nursing education. At its core, simulation is designed to mimic the clinical practice environment by providing students with a realistic experience to apply learned knowledge and skills and by creating a rich learning environment for debriefing and an objective flow of constructive feedback. One type of simulation includes the use of *standardized participants* (SPs) (formerly standardized patients)— individuals trained to act as a real person(s) to simulate a specific situation or clinical experience. Using SPs can be a rich resource for student learning, instruction, practice, and discussion.

Several years ago, I began integrating civility content into my senior level leadership course. I implemented a Problem-Based Learning (PBL) scenario using live actors (SPs) to portray incivility and bullying behaviors among nurses in the workplace. To prepare, students completed reading on the topic of civility and incivility in nursing education and practice. On the day of class, I facilitated an interactive didactic presentation on the topic before the students observed the "live" scenario.

I used three actors to portray a charge nurse and two staff nurses, acting out a situation in which one of the staff nurses was extremely uncivil to her colleagues. The scenario included a nurse manager, Nurse Adams, and Nurse Brown. Nurse Adams was the charge nurse on the evening shift who had always been reliable and professional in her interactions with others. However, lately, Nurse Adams had been consistently late reporting to work and had been isolating herself from others on the unit, which was a distinct change from her previous behavior. The nurse manager had been observing changes in Nurse Adams's behavior, and in that of other staff, which appeared to coincide with the recent hiring of Nurse Brown, an experienced nurse who transferred onto the unit from another department.

When the nurse manager addressed her observations and concerns with Nurse Adams, Nurse Adams first denied any problem. After the nurse manager expressed concern about Nurse Adams's very uncharacteristic behavior and detailed her performance issues, Nurse Adams began to cry and stated, "I just can't stand this anymore." When the nurse manager asked her to explain her comment, Nurse Adams very reluctantly revealed a pattern of abusive behaviors directed toward her by Nurse Brown, including put-downs, negative gossip, intimidating comments, and the withholding of important patient information. When asked why she had not come forward sooner with her complaints, Nurse Adams replied, "I didn't want to be seen as a problem employee."

The nurse manager realized this situation needed to be addressed; however, because she had not witnessed the alleged behaviors, she needed to investigate the situation further. She met privately with Nurse Brown, who did not deny Nurse Adams's report. In fact, she trivialized the situation and sharply stated that Nurse Adams "might be book smart, but she has no common sense, is a big crybaby and needs to toughen up." Nurse Brown was dismissive and curt, and slammed the door on her way out of the nurse manager's office.

After observing the scenario, students analyzed the scenario, developed and practiced specific ways to address the situation, and debriefed the encounter in a large class discussion. I asked students several questions, including:

1. **What was your initial response after witnessing the scenario?**

   Many students commented that Nurse Brown's behavior was offensive, rude, and required supervision and corrective action. The students described Nurse Adams as upset, nervous, submissive, and indicated she was dealing with behaviors frequently occurring in nursing practice. Students also commented on how the scenario allowed them to reflect on their own behaviors, how they might handle the situation, and the way it described how one uncivil person can change an entire culture/environment.

2. **Next, I asked the students how the scenario helped them learn about dealing with incivility in nursing practice.**

   The majority of students believed the role of the nurse manager was important in addressing incivility, and this prompted them to think about how each would handle incivility in practice. The students found the scenario to be realistic, bringing learning "alive," and heightening awareness of incivility and its impact on the practice setting and patient care. Students also noted the importance of teamwork, effective communication, and the need for directed education to address incivility through readings and group discussion.

3. **The next question asked students how the knowledge gained through the learning experience might affect their nursing practice.**

   They commented that the scenario helped them learn how to recognize and address incivility in nursing practice, to be cognizant of their own behavior and how they treat others, to be supportive and respectful, and to effectively communicate. The students also learned that the nurse manager is a valuable resource in managing conflict.

I believe nursing faculty must prepare nursing students to identify and deal with incivility in the practice setting by providing learning experiences to facilitate their transition into the "real world." Nursing students need to be equipped with effective strategies to use if confronted with rude coworkers or belittling supervisors or peers. For more detail about this learning technique, please see Clark, Ahten, and Macy (2014).

I have also incorporated cognitive rehearsal strategies (Griffin, 2004; Griffin & Clark, 2014) for countering uncivil behaviors and empowering new nurses to address and confront instigators and episodes of incivility. After students observe the live PBL scenario, I have them generate and practice specific responses they can use to address uncivil coworkers in the workplace. For example:

> I would like to sit together and have a conversation. I feel that you and I do not understand each other, and it's affecting our work.

> It takes teamwork and support to care for our patients, and your behavior toward me is getting in the way. What can we do to resolve our differences?

> I have noticed a conflict between us, and it is affecting our working relationship and caring for our patients. I would like to discuss the situation and resolve our differences.

I have also asked students to describe specific strategies of how nursing education programs can prepare students to recognize and address incivility in nursing education. Their responses include:

- Integrate civility content throughout the curriculum

- Raise awareness, conduct open forums, and increase education

- Apply active learning strategies (role-play, SPs, case studies, simulation, reflection exercises)

- Practice conflict negotiation, communication, giving and receiving feedback and critique

- Co-create and abide by classroom and clinical norms

- Educate faculty and staff nurses in practice on incivility and fostering civility

- Provide confidential reporting systems; provide "civility liaisons" to assist students in addressing incivility with faculty, nurses in practice, and other students

More recently, I have used a combination of cognitive rehearsal and the TeamSTEPPS's CUS model (Agency for Healthcare Research & Quality [AHRQ], 2016) as a method to equip students with the essential skills needed to effectively address uncivil encounters when they happen, thus increasing the likelihood of success in stopping the behavior and protecting patient safety. Using the uncivil nurse-to-nurse encounter (depicted in the nearby sidebar), students role-play the encounter to simulate real-life experience in addressing incivility. The use of cognitive rehearsal to address incivility generally consists of four parts:

- Participating in didactic instruction

- Learning and rehearsing specific phrases to use during uncivil encounters

- Participating in practice sessions to reinforce instruction and rehearsal of the specific phrases

- De-briefing the uncivil encounters and scripted responses.

CUS, an acronym for Concerned, Uncomfortable, and Safety, is one specific communication structure provided by TeamSTEPPS to assist with conflict negotiation (AHRQ, 2016). I am particularly fond of this model, because students pick up on it quickly and find it helpful in structuring their responses to uncivil and conflicted situations. Following the steps outlined previously, students prepare by reading peer-reviewed works on the topic of civility and incivility in nursing education and practice and by participating in a didactic instruction about the use of cognitive rehearsal and evidence-based frameworks to address uncivil encounters. Next, the students use the CUS model as a structure to frame and practice "scripted" responses to use during uncivil encounters. This step is followed by students participating in or observing the role-played scenario and using their "scripts" to address the situation.

The scenario that I have developed involves two nurses, Carol and Sandy, who work together on a very busy medical surgical unit in a large, major medical center. Carol is exhausted after working three 12-hour shifts in a row and anxious to get home for some much-needed rest after handing off her patient, Mary Jones, to Sandy. Sandy is a few minutes late arriving on the unit. Carol is upset when Sandy arrives and addresses her in a frustrated and irritated manner. Students are asked to role-play (and/or observe) the scenario and respond using a cognitively rehearsed script to address the situation.

> *Geez, Sandy, where have you been? You're late as usual. It's been a really busy shift, and I can't wait to get out of here. See if you can manage to get this information straight for once. You should know Mary Jones by now. You took care of her yesterday, so you should know what's going on. She was on 4S forever. Now she's our problem. She has a bunch of treatments and medications that need to be done. You need to check her vital signs, too. I've been way too busy to do them. So, that's it—I'm out of here. If I forgot something, it's not my problem. Just check the chart.*

Students have enthusiastically embraced this pedagogical approach and have crafted some excellent and effective scripts. Here is one example using the CUS model to frame the response:

> *Carol, I realize being late is not okay, and we can talk about that later if you'd like. For now, I'm Concerned about Mrs. Jones and Uncomfortable rushing through report. For her Safety, please provide a complete report before you go.*

We wrap up the session by de-briefing the uncivil encounters and corresponding responses. Successful de-briefing requires creating safe spaces for reflection and exploring effective ways to address future situations. Examples of de-briefing questions that I have used with success include:

Ask each actor: What was it like to be part of this experience?

Ask observers: What was it like to observe the experience?

Ask actors and observers:

How would you describe the experience?

What went well? What would you do again?

What did you/we learn? What might be done differently next time?

Semester after semester, student feedback reveals a vital need to integrate civility content into courses and, more importantly, throughout the curriculum.

Teaching in the Online Learning Environment

Dr. Lori Candela is a gifted nursing professor with decades of experience teaching in both in-class and online learning environments. Her masterful and deep descriptions of learning theories and frameworks to guide faculty in the online teaching-learning experience are excellent. As such, I asked Lori to contribute to this section. In Chapter 4, I provided a brief description of online learning in higher education in general and nursing education in particular and noted that enrollment in online classes will continue to grow. By 2013, the number of college students taking at least one online course soared to 7.1 million (Huss, Sela, & Eastep, 2015), representing 32% of all college students (Younger & Ahern, 2015). The movement toward online offerings is also apparent in nursing programs. Many nursing programs offer graduate programs and RN-to-BSN programs that are delivered completely online. More and more undergraduate nursing programs are converting selected face to face (F2F) courses to online and/or using a blended format in which some portions of the course are delivered online and some are provided F2F. Successful online courses rely on creating and nurturing an engaged, civil community of learners. Like incivility that may be seen in F2F classrooms, incivility may also occur in the online learning environment, which can take the form of posting rumors or misinformation, gossiping, or publishing materials that defame and humiliate others.

The online learning environment can be stressful for both students and faculty. Dacanay, Vaughn, Orr, Andre, and Mort (2015) found that students enrolled in an online RN-to-BSN program indicated a need for more opportunities to be connected and to have consistent support and feedback from faculty. Both can be a challenge in online courses. The real-time communication used in F2F courses provides opportunities to promptly adjust content based on student understanding of the course material and to immediately address uncivil behaviors. Making these adjustments is more difficult in an online environment. Interactions are often asynchronous and do not offer the ability to "read" another individual based on facial expression or body posture (Smith, 2005). There is also a transactional distance, a cognitive space between educators and learners (Huss et al., 2015) that can result in frustration, anxiety, and even anger. Because students often sit alone in front of their laptops or computers, they can often feel isolated and disconnected. These conditions can be fertile ground for uncivil online behaviors.

Unlike the F2F classroom, all or nearly all of the communication in online courses occurs by written communication. This style of communication may lead to an "impersonal milieu," which may contribute to casual types of communication that may be perceived as offensive, challenging, harassing, belittling, demanding, or even hostile (Galbraith & Jones, 2010). Other students may be disengaged, withdrawn, or non-responsive, which may also be perceived as uncivil or discourteous, particularly if they are working in groups. Faculty may also be perceived as uncaring and/or failing to engage students by not being "present" in the course (Huss et al., 2015).

The Community of Inquiry (CoI) model is a helpful way to promote learning, engagement, and connection in an online learning environment. The CoI focuses on three main areas of presence to enhance the learning experience:

1. Teaching presence (interaction with teacher via course structure and process),

2. Cognitive presence (content interaction), and

3. Social presence (peer interaction),

in order to establish a sense of community, respect, and responsibility (Garrison & Akyol, 2013). Mayne and Wu (2011) suggested that social presence is among the most significant factors in promoting connectedness and a sense of community. It can decrease the sense of being alone in the course. Social interaction combined with shared learning goals helps to promote good course citizenship (Bonnel & Vogel Smith, 2010). The teaching presence in the CoI is integral in both setting the climate and interacting during the course in ways that role-model the caring, supportive behaviors displayed by teachers every day in F2F classrooms.

To promote a civil online learning environment, educators should include clear and complete content with exemplars that are aligned with the learning objectives and evaluations. Courses should be logical in flow and easy to navigate. The course syllabus should include clear, detailed explanations of strategies for being successful in the online learning environment, student and faculty expectations, and how that course content will be delivered and evaluated.

Clarity, transparency, and consistency are important in all aspects of the online course. Students should know what the turnaround time is for getting email queries answered and for assignments to be returned. Evaluation rubrics should be detailed and clear. Students often work in groups to complete assignments. It can be very helpful to start each group off with a phone or online meeting to discuss how the group will work together and how issues will be handled. This is an opportune time to clarify any questions about assignments. It may also be helpful to provide exemplar papers and exemplar discussion pages so students can get a better sense of what high-quality work looks like.

Like the "live" classroom, the first week in the online course should be used to co-create class norms to promote a civil learning environment. Here is an exemplar for co-creating norms:

During the first week of the course:

1. *Assemble students into small groups.*

2. *Ask each group member to identify 5–10 behaviors (norms) expected to be followed by each member of the group in the online course. These behaviors are designed to foster a civil learning environment, promote learning and support for one another, and describe how uncivil behaviors will be addressed if the norms are not followed.*

3. *Have each group member post their list of norms and corresponding consequences to the discussion board.*

4. *Ask each group to develop a final, agreed-upon list of norms with ways to address the situation if norms are not followed.*

5. *Once all students agree to the norms and corresponding consequences, post the list on the online course site for easy reference.*

6. *Keep the list front and center throughout the semester.*

Clearly, the appeal of online learning has increased dramatically among nursing students. Simultaneously, the rise of popularity for online learning has created potential avenues for uncivil behaviors that can affect student satisfaction, performance, and retention. For a detailed description of a mixed-methodological study on cyberbullying and online incivility in nursing education, see the two-part article series published in *Nurse Educator* (Clark, Ahten, & Werth, 2012; Clark, Werth, & Ahten, 2012).

Faculty must design realistic and relevant learning activities that represent actual practice as closely as possible. Because conflict among nurses is a significant issue resulting in job dissatisfaction, absenteeism, and turnover (Almost, 2006), Candela uses a conflict experience to engage online learners. She uses students' own experiences with work situations that involve conflict. The conflict provides the context to facilitate learning through reflection, sharing, and understanding from peer perspectives. The steps in the nearby sidebar are used to develop and implement the teaching strategy.

USING CONFLICT EXPERIENCES TO ENGAGE ONLINE LEARNERS

DR. LORI CANDELA

1. *The students are randomly assigned into groups of three when the course opens.*

2. *They are informed at the beginning of the course (via syllabus and orientation video) about a small-group course assignment involving two, synchronous, 1-hour calls.*

continues

continued

3. The instructor sets up call times that are convenient for each group via their small-group discussion area and the preferred format (telephone conference or Skype).

4. Several weeks before the call, the instructor emails instructions for preparation and participation to student groups, along with the evaluation rubric. Additionally, background information on conflict as a learning opportunity, relationship building, whole listening, and asking questions for understanding is provided in each small-group discussion area.

5. Student preparation for the call involves reflecting on a conflict situation from work that you have been directly involved in that made (or makes) you uncomfortable.

6. Students are sent reminders during the semester of upcoming calls.

7. During the call, the instructor acts as call facilitator and timekeeper.

8. The format for the call and procedures for maintaining privacy and confidentiality (not identifying others or workplaces by name) are briefly reviewed at the beginning of each call.

9. A round of thought-provoking questions is facilitated to explore perceptions of conflict in general.

10. Each student shares a conflict situation, emotions that came up, how it was handled, what the relationships are like now with the people who were involved in the conflict, and how the student feels about it now.

11. Group members ask additional questions to further understand the conflict.

12. Group members then provide alternative ways to look at the situation and work with others to resolve the issue while nurturing relationships.

13. The call is summarized by asking each student to reflect on what they learned and how they will use it.

14. Students are invited to provide any additional feedback or suggestions via the course website.

Candela reports that several students have provided positive comments about the calls, including developing their abilities to be fully present to others, communicate through listening and asking questions, learning to see conflicts as opportunities to build and sustain work relationships, and the value of seeking the perspective of others.

Mastering Our Craft

Faculty who intentionally focus on mastering the art of teaching will surely experience fewer problems with disruptive student behavior. As my friend Dr. Luparell puts it, "Students do not deserve an 'A' merely because they pay tuition; however, students do deserve to get the product they pay for, and in academics that means quality instruction. Thus, faculty who wish to have better relationships with students absolutely must attend to their craft as a priority." I couldn't agree more. Many excellent sources can improve our teaching acumen, and many colleges and universities have a center for teaching and learning—all of these can be helpful to both novice and seasoned educators.

A few semesters ago, I contacted the director of our center for teaching and learning and asked her for a list of 10 to 12 faculty whom she considered to be highly skilled teachers within our university. I contacted five or six of the professors on the list, choosing them from a broad range of disciplines and class sizes, and asked each one if I could visit their classroom, observe their teaching and learning techniques, and engage in a conversation with them following my experience. All of them agreed.

One of my favorite experiences involved the observation of a social science professor who facilitated a class of more than 250 students. The large traditional lecture hall consists of row after row of wooden seats with built-in writing tables that extend from floor to ceiling. This environment is not necessarily conducive to engaged learning. Yet, despite the structure and size of the classroom, this masterful teacher created an incredible learning experience for his students. Using PowerPoint slides, he projected large, colorful images of events that related to the class content. The slides included no text; there were simply amazing images that led to spirited discussion and free exchange of ideas and social discourse about the history and politics of the time. Even more amazing was the professor's ability to address his students by name. Given the size of the class, this was an astounding accomplishment.

Later, when we met over coffee to discuss my observations and to probe his teaching strategies, he revealed his secret to learning the names of so many students. At the beginning of each semester, he uses a university web-based system to download a color copy of each student's photo with associated information such as name, major, and year in school. He places the photo on a 3x5 index card and takes them to each class to begin to associate names with faces. He also invites students to meet with him at least once a semester so that he can get to know them a little bit better. It is not required, but the professor offers a few extra credit points for students who take him up on his offer. When the student makes an appointment, the professor has the card ready to again associate the photo the person—and makes notes on the card highlighting key points of the meeting.

Yes, this technique takes time, but according to the professor, it is well worth it. Students feel valued and respected, and classroom incivility is almost nonexistent. What a wonderful experience for the students, the professor, and for me—to be given such a rich experience to attend this class and learn from a master! I have learned so much from my observational experiences that I continue to visit other professors' classrooms and invite them to observe mine.

Finding Your "Unique Voice"

Finding and celebrating your passion for teaching and expressing your "unique voice" helps to keep your enthusiasm for teaching alive. In the preceding section, I described my practice of visiting other professors' classrooms to enhance my own teaching and to learn fresh approaches to fostering student learning. One day, I was visiting the classroom of one of our gifted history professors. It was a beautiful spring day. As I walked across the campus quad and neared the lecture hall, I was immediately surrounded by the invigorating and nostalgic sound of World War II music. Upon entering the classroom, I noticed some students taking their seats, others visiting with the professor, and most enjoying the music. When it was time for class, the professor turned off the recording and spent the first 10 minutes discussing how the music of an era provides a window into a historic time. The conversation was spectacular! Later, when we met to discuss my observations of her class, I asked about the use of music. She was thoughtful for a moment, and then said, "Music is my passion—it inspires me to inspire my students."

Clearly this talented professor had found her "unique voice" to ignite her teaching passion. This conversation encouraged me to discover my "unique voice." What is it that makes my teaching special or unique? What is a distinguishing characteristic of my teaching? What inspires me to inspire my students? It didn't take long for me to realize what it is about my teaching that makes it unique. I love the art and practice of storytelling—weaving and sharing a personal yarn or threading a funny or poignant anecdote into the topic of the day. Most of the time, the stories are based on my own experiences, but other times, I read a passage from a classic or a book that illuminates and amplifies the subject matter. I have a deep passion for books; I love the feel and smell of an old tome, cracking the binding and turning the pages to discover an unlimited galaxy of possibilities, understanding, and expanded thinking, experiencing an incredible intellectual or entertaining journey taking me anywhere my mind can travel. I have a vast collection of books, and each class period I bring at least one (sometimes several) to class and encourage my students to add them to their reading "wish list" and to peruse them when time and space allows. My students have come to enjoy the books that I carry into my classroom nestled in a beautiful basket—a receptacle worthy of such treasures.

So, think about what makes you and your teaching extraordinary. What ignites your passion? How might you pass this passion onto your students? Take time to reflect, and after you realize and discover your "unique voice," share it boldly, broadly, and with the passion it deserves!

Finishing Touches

Faculty play a key role in creating and sustaining positive student-faculty relationships through learning experiences that promote collaborative exchanges between students and faculty. Active learning strategies not only promote student achievement and productivity, they minimize disruption and reduce the potential for incivility by promoting cooperation, collaboration, and student engagement. Active learning techniques can also be used to provide students with an understanding of incivility and its impact on the practice setting, including ways to prevent and address uncivil behavior. Many of my students have reported a favorable reaction to my use of these active learning strategies, a heightened awareness of incivility in nursing practice, and an increased level of confidence in their abilities to address uncivil behaviors in their future workplaces.

CIVILITY TIP

Make it a priority to get students involved with their own learning experience—give them an assignment ahead of time, arrange them in groups (or better yet, have them self-arrange), ask students to reflect on their assignment and to share their "gems" and "pearls" of discovery and enlightenment. By having written assignments discussed in small groups, you can increase discussion and class participation and encourage quiet students to add their ideas at their own pace.

Chapter 11
The Healing Power of Stress Management and Self-Care

Incivility exacts an emotional toll and zaps our energy—so we must take care of ourselves, nurture the spirit, and create a healing milieu.
–Cynthia Clark

This chapter discusses:

- Recognizing the signs of stress and burnout
- Engaging in self-care strategies
- Living in gratitude

Eustress and Not-So-Eustress

As a young undergraduate student, in addition to pursuing my bachelor's degree, I was also seeking minor degrees in psychology and sociology. I remember very clearly taking a course on the relationship between stress and mental health. The professor discussed a type of positive stress called "eustress" that prepares us for immediate action, increases creativity, and arises when we need inspiration and motivation. We learned that some stress can be beneficial and create feelings of well-being and fulfillment, assuming the individual perceives the event as positive.

Ultimately, perceptions of any event, including uncivil encounters, are open to individual interpretation. In other words, behavior that might be perceived as uncivil by one person might not be perceived the same way by another. Each person perceives and interprets these interactions within the context of his or her personal experiences and through the lens of his or her own worldview. If a person perceives or experiences a behavior as uncivil, stress can manifest in unhealthy ways. Many factors influence the perceptions of civility and incivility including the intent of the behavior; the context in which the behavior occurs; and the attitudes, values, and beliefs held by the recipient of the behavior (Clark & Carnosso, 2008). In other words, incivility often exists in the "eye of the beholder" and is affected by cultural issues, real or perceived power differences, and varying perceptions of what constitutes uncivil behavior.

Whether intended or not, the impact of incivility can be quite stressful. Very real physiological changes occur in response to stress. Cortisol is a steroid hormone controlled by the pituitary gland, produced in the cortex of the adrenal glands, and essential to energy regulation and mobilization. When a person is stressed, cortisol, epinephrine, and norepinephrine are released from the adrenal glands, resulting in a "stress reaction." Initially, our immune system will protect us during stressful times; however, chronic stress causes a decrease in immunologic protection. We begin to experience the flu, colds, skin breakouts, stomach aches, and infections. The continuous release of cortisol has been linked to abdominal obesity (belly fat) and associated with overeating and craving fatty and sugary foods. The stress reaction also causes an increase in heart rate and blood pressure, and when stress is prolonged and recovery from it seems hopeless, the individual might become depleted and discouraged.

Obviously, stress will always be a part of our lives, and mild stress levels can give us an edge. However, too much stress, especially if prolonged and coupled with poor coping habits, might cause physical, emotional, and spiritual fatigue and ill health. Chronic stress plays a role in developing type 2 diabetes, cardiovascular disease, and mental illness. Self-care and stress-management strategies are important for managing stress and lessening the health risks associated with chronic stress. Carol Shively, pathology professor at Wake Forest University School of Medicine, states that stress management "might be the one weight-loss strategy that society hasn't really addressed" (Parker-Pope, 2005, p. 1).

Signs of Stress and Burnout

Various signs and symptoms point to stress and burnout. I have included some common ones in the following list, though I am sure you can easily add to them:

- Belly fat
- Insomnia
- Fatigue
- Irritability and anger
- Lack of interest
- Depression
- Headaches
- Muscular tension
- Appetite changes
- Stomach aches
- Intestinal problems
- Frequent colds, flu, and infection
- Nervousness
- Excessive worry
- Lost time with friends and loved ones

Let's take a closer look at various types of stress—for example, *job stress* is defined as a feeling that one's capabilities, resources, or needs do not match the demands of the job. Heavy and/or inequitable workloads, communication problems, conflicted work environments, unfair compensation, and keeping up with technology changes are some sources of job stress. Other sources of job stress include job reassignment, loss of position or status, inability to retire when desired, and a lack of job security. According to the 2015 *Stress in America* report (American Psychological Association [APA], 2015), job stress is the second most common source of stress among U.S. adults, just behind stress caused by money and financial concerns. And 60% of adults say their jobs are a somewhat significant or very significant source of stress. When stress levels mount, burnout may occur. The Mayo Clinic (2015) defines *burnout* as a special type of job stress—a state of physical, emotional, or mental exhaustion combined with doubts about your competence and the value of your work. Their newsletter provides a set of questions to assess your level of potential burnout.

Ask yourself the following questions (Mayo Clinic, 2015):

1. Have you become cynical or critical at work?

2. Do you drag yourself to work and have trouble getting started once you arrive?

3. Have you become irritable or impatient with coworkers, customers, or clients?

4. Do you lack the energy to be consistently productive?

5. Do you lack satisfaction from your achievements?

6. Do you feel disillusioned about your job?

7. Are you using food, drugs, or alcohol to feel better or to simply not feel?

8. Have your sleep habits or appetite changed?

9. Are you troubled by unexplained headaches, backaches, or other physical complaints?

The Mayo Clinic newsletter's advice: "If you answered yes to any of these questions, you may be experiencing job burnout. Be sure to consult your doctor or a mental health provider, however. Some of these symptoms can also indicate certain health conditions, such as a thyroid disorder or depression" (Mayo Clinic, 2015, p. 2).

Job burnout can result from various factors, including a lack of control over your schedule, assignments, or workload; unclear job expectations; mismatched personal and organizational values; poor job fit; or an uncivil workplace (Mayo Clinic, 2015). I have listed several signs of burnout here—how do you fare?

- Workaholism
- Chronic fatigue
- Not wanting to go to work

- Increase in sick time

- Negative attitude

- Blaming and criticizing others

- Engaging in backbiting

- Marginalizing others

- Talking behind others' backs, gossiping

Strategies for Self-Care and Stress Management

Because stress is a reality of life, and eliminating it is impossible, we all need to know and practice a variety of stress-management techniques. As I reflect on my life, I have consistently used various stress-management strategies—many of them physical.

As an adult, I started kickboxing. Under the tutelage of my sensei of more than 15 years, I learned the importance of discipline, commitment to hard work, and training my mind and body to react and defend. The cardio-kickboxing classes were intense; kicking and punching heavy bags was physical and grueling. Some days the clock seemed to stand still as I ran, punched, kicked, and performed countless plyometric and boxing drills—and then did it all over again. Things do not always go well in the dojo and in studying the martial arts; I've been knocked down, bruised, and had surgery on my shoulder and knee because I stubbornly refused to back down from a much stronger, bigger, and quicker opponent. I have learned from my mistakes, learned how to get back up and how to keep fighting the good fight. Most of all, I think I have learned that family, friends, and people matter—that life is short, that we are all in it together, and that the people we meet along life's journey enrich and inform our lives. I have learned and experienced firsthand the power of kinship, companionship, and fellowship. I have also experienced fierceness juxtaposed with surprising tenderness and grace. Just like the physical muscle memory I have developed and honed, I have also strengthened my mental muscle memory for restraint, respect, and civility. Life in the dojo transcended the physical—it has increased my capacity for awareness, mental fitness, and moral courage. Perhaps someday, I will hang up my boxing gloves, but for now, the scent of sweat and leather and the crisp smack of my gloves beckon.

Kickboxing is a total body, mind, and spirit experience. In our dojo, the punching, kicking, highly charged cardio workouts are embedded in the tenets of the martial arts, where the sensei reinforces important daily and relevant life lessons. In the accompanying sidebar, I describe some of the benefits of kickboxing and its influence on building my civility competence.

LESSONS FROM THE DOJO

Kickboxing improves my:

- *Ability to predict troublesome situations*
- *Capacity to protect myself from real or potential danger*
- *Outlook on life*
- *Respect for myself and others*
- *Level of alertness and awareness of others and my surroundings*
- *Confidence and self-esteem*
- *Physical, mental, and spiritual strength*
- *Stress-management and self-care capacity*
- *Fitness, balance, and mental acuity*
- *Self-discipline, self-control, and character*
- *Ability to "read" people and anticipate their actions and reactions*

What are your stress reducers? Take a minute to jot down your favorite stress-busters and share them with a friend. Identifying and sticking with the stress-reducing techniques that work for you is vital. Several types of exercises and activities are effective in reducing or managing stress. I mentioned my love for cardio-kickboxing, but less intense, gentler exercise programs, such as Pilates, yoga, and tai chi can work as well. Meditation, progressive relaxation, deep breathing, and visualization are other methods that can be effective in decreasing stress-induced symptoms. Also, eating right and getting enough rest should be incorporated in a stress-management plan for life.

Putting Self-Care on Your Schedule

Years ago, when our children were younger, my husband and I were so busy juggling and managing their activities that I found little time for myself. One of the best pieces of advice I received was to enter my workouts and "me time" into my calendar and treat them as importantly as any other work meeting or children's activity. At first, it was challenging to put my "time" into my calendar, but it was so effective that I still use this method today. By taking care of myself, I can better attend to the needs of others. In fact, I was recently asked to schedule a meeting with a colleague; she suggested a particular date and time, and when I checked my calendar, I noted that I was scheduled for my weight-lifting class during the suggested time. I offered an alternative meeting date and time that worked well for my colleague and that did not interfere with my workout. It was a win-win situation!

When I think about the power of self-care, I am reminded of a compelling story related by Dr. Regina Benjamin, U.S. Surgeon General, during her 2011 keynote address at a national nursing conference. Benjamin is an amazing physician and national leader who has emphasized the importance of self-care so that we might better attend to the care of others. In her role as Surgeon General, Benjamin traveled frequently by air. Many of us who fly often are keenly familiar with the flight attendants' instructions about safety measures. However, often we tune them out, read our book, listen to our iPods, or fall asleep as we prepare for takeoff. Benjamin often did the same; however, one day she decided to focus on the details of the safety instructions. When the flight attendant reminded the passengers, "In the event of an emergency, cabin pressure will change and oxygen masks will drop, be sure to put your own mask on first, before placing it on children or other compromised individuals," Benjamin took notice. You see, to nurses and doctors, this advice might seem counterintuitive, because we are caregivers and unused to doing for ourselves before doing for others. But that is the power of Benjamin's story—each of us needs to take good personal self-care to be at full capacity to help others. This message reinforced a valuable lesson I learned in graduate school while studying to be an adolescent and family therapist. Our professors emphasized that for children to be healthy, the parental unit needed to be strong and enduring. They stressed the importance of a united parental relationship, and for parents to take care of themselves individually and together to provide the best possible foundation for their children to thrive. Once again, though it seems somewhat counterintuitive, parents must focus on their connection to role-model safe, supportive, and healthy relationships. When children witness genuine love and mutual respect, they are likely to flourish. This role-modeling of civility will help promote civil behavior in the future.

Fostering Gratitude

I am also a big fan of gratitude journals. I can remember with extreme clarity when I learned the value and the power of focusing on the things in life for which we are truly grateful. More than a dozen years ago, my husband traveled on an extensive trip with his brother and two friends to a very remote area in Alaska. It was before cellphones, and because he had no access to a landline, I would be completely isolated from my husband for nearly 3 weeks. Though I appreciated his need to travel for an extended time with his brother and friends, I was frustrated to be left alone to care for our three young children. I could not relate to my husband's need to be away, nor could I comprehend being so completely isolated from my children and the rest of the world. In an effort to understand, I asked my husband to explain his fascination with needing to get away and experience nature, its marvels, and maybe even its dangers. He told me that communing with nature and being completely away helped him reconnect with his spirituality, refueled and reenergized him, and strengthened his love for me and the children. I tried to understand, but regrettably, I was so focused on my own "issues" that I failed to appreciate his. Blame it on youth or immaturity, but it was not until I went for a long run with my best friend that I finally got it. During our run, I explained my frustration with my husband being gone. My friend is a great listener and also very honest. She took note, paid attention, and listened politely. She has known my husband for a very long time and knows what a wonderful man he is, so she asked, "Cindy, why are you being so selfish? Why are you so focused on the 2% of your relationship that bothers you instead of the 98% that you love and appreciate about your husband?" She chided and reminded me that my husband is a loving, devoted, giving father, husband, and friend. She encouraged me to let go of the anger and find the gratitude. What a shocker! I was stunned. My friend was not validating my position; instead she questioned my focus. It took some time, but very soon, I realized she was spot-on.

After the run, I could not get our conversation out of my head. I knew that my husband would continue his trips, and accepting this was important to our lives together. The following day, I was watching a television program and suddenly had an epiphany. The program was about the power of gratitude and being grateful instead of resentful. So there it was again, another example of what I had been doing in my own life, focusing on what was wrong instead of what was positive. At that very moment, the cloud lifted and my thoughts became much clearer. The program host suggested that viewers list at least five things for which they are grateful each day. As soon as the show ended, I grabbed a journal and wrote down five things for which I am grateful:

1. My husband and our children

2. Good friends

3. Cool cloud cover on a 100° day

4. Good books by amazing authors

5. The sound and smell of a fresh rainfall

Today I wrote:

1. Flights that depart and arrive on time

2. Cool morning hikes with our merry band of rescue pets

3. Bold, rich coffee served in my favorite mug

4. Bike rides on country roads outside our Boise home

5. Waking to the sound of mourning doves, meadowlarks, and other desert songbirds

Focusing on gratitude, appreciation, and love for the people and things around us can help decrease stress and put life into perspective. In his book titled *Spontaneous Happiness,* Dr. Andrew Weil (2011) describes keeping a gratitude journal as a means to boost happiness levels. Weil suggests devoting a few minutes each day to give thanks for the good things in our lives and counting our blessings. Expressing gratitude might be one of the most effective strategies in achieving and maintaining a contented life. Forgiveness is a close cousin to gratitude and another important key to emotional health. Both must be practiced on a daily basis.

In my role as a consultant, I meet many administrators, faculty, students, nurses, and other healthcare workers from around the country. I am constantly amazed at their high levels of stress. I recall meeting with a group of approximately 15 university deans from a large institution to discuss strategies to improve the academic work environment. We were scheduled for a 2-hour session, and my plan was to present a brief formal presentation before opening the meeting to questions and strategic dialogue. We were just about to begin—my slides and handouts at the ready—when I decided to approach the session in a different way. As I looked around the room, I sensed a heightened level of stress and anxiety; so, on impulse, I made a quick decision to open the meeting with a question. After brief introductions, I asked them, "Tell me what it's like to be a dean. How do you spend your days?"

The entire room fell silent—you could have heard a pin drop. At first, I worried that I had asked a question that might be deemed too personal Then one by one, several individuals opened up and talked about their lives. One commented, "You don't know me, but I have gained 40 pounds in the 2 years since I became a dean. My stress level is off the charts; I eat too much, and many of my food choices are unhealthy. I'm pretty miserable." Another stated, "I'm divorced; this job is all-consuming and my wife simply got tired of being alone." Another commented, "I miss teaching and contact with students; it seems that I spend my days putting out fires, dealing with conflict, and managing difficult people. It's exhausting." A few others sat quietly, and I learned later in the meeting that they were new to their role as dean. I hoped that they would be OK. We discussed the importance of self-care and engaging in stress-reducing activities. It's challenging enough to transform a work environment in the best of circumstances, but when we are stressed—or worse, approaching burnout—change seems almost impossible.

Chatting with the deans reminded me of my many conversations with faculty; it's simply a variation on the theme. I recall a nursing professor commenting, "It's only the first month of classes, and I am completely exhausted. I'm teaching two 12-hour clinical days and an extra class as an overload assignment because we have unfilled faculty positions, and there is no one else to teach the class. I'm also enrolled in a DNP program, because our university requires all faculty members to obtain a doctoral degree. We have a new director, and she has asked me to take on some of the school's administrative responsibilities, which I have agreed to do. On top of everything, our current cohort of students is more challenging than ever, and I am completely drained."

Concerned for her, I asked: "What are you doing for yourself?"

She looked at me with a resigned expression and said, "To be perfectly honest, I am doing very little, if anything, to nurture myself. I'm just too busy."

Nurturing Body, Mind, and Soul

Unfortunately, these stories are not uncommon. And, when I ask others what they are doing to nurture themselves, sadly, the vast majority say they are working so hard and moving in so many directions that self-care has taken a back seat to responsibilities that often overwhelm them.

This is deeply concerning because lack of self-care takes a significant toll on personal, physical, emotional, and spiritual well-being, and it can have a potentially negative impact on our ability to care for others, including patients. The pressure created by competing demands from family, work, and life responsibilities can cause stress and maybe even burnout.

Living in gratitude, keeping a journal, and honoring "me time" activities are important steps toward self-care, yet there are other effective ways to manage stress. In my opinion, real and lasting change comes from identifying the sources of our stress and creating an intentional plan to deal with them. Consider carrying a small notebook or make a note using your smartphone to record events or situations that cause you stress. After a week or two, you will likely gain a clear picture of where your stress is coming from and how you might address it.

Once you've made a personal list of stressors, identify those that you can do something about and those that are out of your control.

For example, you may be stressed by your work commute. Is there a way to change the method, timing, or route of your commute to reduce your stress? If so, this is something within your control. If you identify a stressor that you cannot effectively eliminate—for example, caring for a young child or a family member living with a disability—think about ways to reduce the stress involved. Are there other people or community resources available that can share your care responsibilities and thereby lessen your stress?

Regardless of the sources of your stress or whether you can change them, putting yourself first is essential. This is not a selfish endeavor. By taking care of yourself, you can better attend to the needs of others. Some of us benefit from physical exercise and activities such as yoga, meditation, progressive relaxation, deep breathing, and enjoying music or the outdoors. Spending time with family, friends, and pets; eating nutritious foods; and getting enough rest also help reduce stress.

Managing your time well and staying organized can also be stress-reducing. Start each day with a "to-do" list and arrange them by priority, from high to low. Consider dropping low-priority tasks altogether by rescheduling them for completion sometime in the future, or better yet, when possible, delegate those tasks to someone else. Resist multitasking and the urge to immediately respond to every text or email message you receive. Prioritize the messages, and, if possible, save them to a folder to be addressed when you have more time.

"Unplug" from your phone, television, computer, and other distractions to enjoy a moment of peace and quiet. Take a deep breath, and clear your mind. When life is busy, we often get distracted and lose connection with those we care about most. Schedule a date night with your partner, enjoy lunch or a power walk with a friend, or spend time with your furry friends. Avoid negative people as much as possible, and surround yourself with those who bring fun and laughter into your life. Take time off, or schedule a mini-vacation. Whatever you decide to do to de-stress, remember, you deserve it!

Although eliminating stress is impossible, minimizing it and engaging in self-care techniques can be extremely helpful and ultimately important in achieving an overall state of wellness. So, take a minute to jot down your favorite stress-busters and most effective stress-reducing techniques and weave them into the daily fabric of your life. At times, we need to de-stress "in the moment" and engage in just-in-time (JiT) techniques to decrease stress in the here and now. Here are a few suggestions.

First, try progressive relaxation—start by tensing and releasing each muscle group in your body beginning from your head down to your toes; start with your facial muscles, then flow to your neck, arms, torso, abdomen, legs, all the way down to your toes. Use a combination of deep breathing, stretching, and positive visualization. As you breathe deeply, stand on your tiptoes, extend your hands over your head, and reach with your fingers as far as you're able toward the ceiling. As you are deep breathing and stretching, imagine a calm and peaceful scene and repeat a positive affirmation such as *"Stress is leaving my body; my work is very important; I am making a positive difference in the lives of my patients; what I do matters."*

As a teacher, I specifically addressed self-care and stress management with my nursing students. We discussed helpful techniques and ways to reduce stress "in the moment" and beyond. I frequently invited my colleague Marty Downey, PhD, RN, AHN-BC, HTPA (holistic nurse extraordinaire), to facilitate class and engage the students (and me) in various self-care and stress-management exercises. I have included several of Dr. Downey's strategies in the sidebars that follow. I know you and your colleagues and students will find them helpful.

According to Downey, nurses, nurse educators, nurse leaders, and nursing students at all levels are surrounded by life events or stressors that stretch our mind-body-spirit resources, and if the demand is higher than the supply of resources, stress is the result. Managing stress and creating balance are significant for all nurses. Learning relaxation techniques, such as imagery, massage, energy repatterning, and sense therapies, can assist nurses in meeting daily goals of maintaining and enhancing physical, mental, and spiritual health. Personal use of complementary therapies (CT) expands the nurse's knowledge base for professional practice (Downey, 2006). Nurses who develop a self-healthcare plan integrating mind-body-spirit rituals for increasing energy and maintaining balance in their lives are more effective care providers. The sidebars at the end of this chapter cover a few simple steps that can bring a sense of peace and calm during stressful moments and challenging times.

NOTE

Complementary therapies are also called alternative or holistic therapies and might include such techniques as aromatherapy, herbal medicine, guided imagery, and yoga.

HAND MASSAGE

DR. MARTY DOWNEY

1. *First, always ask permission of the patient/client.*

2. *The provider (you) should wash hands in warm water and dry hands prior to touching the patient's hands.*

3. *Offer your hand and the client will offer his or hers.*

4. *Place a small dollop of hand lotion on the patient's hand. Use a scented lotion if the patient is not allergic to scented lotions, preferably scented with lavender.*

5. *With the patient's palm facing down, gently stretch the patient's hand out by spreading the palm open, using your fingers from underneath.*

6. *Make small circles with your thumbs on top of the patient's hand moving up to the wrist.*

7. *Massage along the web spaces starting at the wrist and moving toward the fingertips.*

8. *Press down between the bones on the soft tissue, not on the bones. Apply generous pressure and check that it is not too much. Do this a couple of times along each web space.*

9. *Turn the patient's hand over and stretch it out again by spreading the palm apart with your thumbs.*

10. *Smooth out the palm and then separate the fingers with your own fingers.*

11. *Make small circles over the whole palm from wrist to fingers, again applying generous pressure and paying special attention to the thumb and joints at the base of the thumb.*

12. *Bring the attention to the fingers: Squeeze and gently twist each finger from base to nail.*

    a. *Start by squeezing along the sides.*

    b. *Next, press and wring along the top and bottom.*

    c. *Then pull gently on the finger when you get to the tip of the finger.*

    d. *Repeat this process for each finger.*

Replicate the entire massage on the other hand.

PROGRESSIVE RELAXATION EXERCISE

DR. MARTY DOWNEY

For this exercise to be effective, the participants need to set aside 20–30 minutes of quiet. If you would like to use this as a relaxation session for yourself and others, you could make a recording of this session/exercise, adding background music for easy listening. The leader could also provide a podcast.

In a quiet, comfortable (temperature) environment with dim lighting, lie or sit on a soothing surface. When you or your patient/client is ready, begin the progressive relaxation exercise:

Prepare yourself and allow your eyes to close softly. Center yourself by focusing on the rhythm and feel of your breathing. Breathe deeply through your nose and slowly allow the air to flow out through your lips. Breathe deeply for three cycles; then turn your attention to areas of tension in your body. Become aware of any tension that you might feel in your scalp and forehead. Take a slow breath and, while slowly releasing your breath, release the tension in your scalp and forehead. Become

continues

continued

attentive to strain in your face, lips, mouth, and tongue. Slowly breathe in and out while softening skin and muscles in these areas. Moving your focus to your neck and throat, feel a sense of release, warmth, and relaxation spreading down the neck and throat to your shoulders, upper back, and upper arms, as if a warm blue blanket has been placed across your shoulders. Release any tension in this area as you take a deep breath, relaxing these muscles. Spread this wave of relaxation down to your arms, (breathe) forearms, and hands (breathe). Release tension through your hands and fingers. You could even shake your hands gently to release the tension out the tips of the fingers. Slowly breathe in and out, and then focus your attention on your chest and upper back. With a deep breath, let go of any tension and spread this relaxation down through your abdomen. Take a moment, and then release that relaxation to your mid- and lower back. Free the pressure, allowing relaxation as you breathe.

As you bring your attention to the lower part of your torso, smooth any tension that you hold in your pelvic area, buttocks, and thighs. Release and smooth the muscles of the lower limbs. Continue to breathe slowly, deeply, and fully.

This relaxation will continue to bring your attention to your calves and feet. Send the smoothing sensation to the feet and out the toes, pretending that you are planting your feet in warm, comfortable earth. Send your roots into the earth as it takes up the tension and brings a sense of calm up through the roots into your muscles, relaxing your body, mind, and spirit.

Rest in this position and allow your mind to create a memory for this relaxed feeling. Your breathing is relaxed, and you are in a place of deep relaxation. When you create this memory, you are able to give yourself permission to bring this feeling to your mind, body, and spirit whenever you feel stressed or tense. Quickly and easily, this thought of relaxation will stimulate a physical response to the mind's request.

At the right moment, breathe deeply; bring your consciousness to the environment that you are in right now. It is safe and calm. Slowly open your eyes, extend your arms above your head or out to the sides, wiggle your fingers and toes, breathe, and return to the environment with a sense of renewed energy and repose.

GUIDED IMAGERY SCENARIO
DR. MARTY DOWNEY

This session can take approximately 10–20 minutes, so allow time and create space in a warm, quiet, comfortable environment. For the auditory sense, add music if you or the client is open to this. Place an intention/goal for the session. Perhaps you need pain relief or balance or simple relaxation. Say this out loud. Then, begin to assess yourself or the client by asking him or her to describe a favorite place of relaxation and repose. Be sure to include all of the sensory fine points of the chosen environment: An image of the ocean would include the beach sounds, the feel of the breeze, the temperature of the surrounding area, and the aromas. You will know when to continue as you or the client begins to relax in a comfortable position. Soften your voice, slowly and with pauses between breaths, and say the following script:

Allow your attention to match the rhythm of your breathing. Breathing slowly in and out, create an image of a comfortable setting. In this setting, a sense of peace and calm surrounds you. Bring to mind the colors of the setting (pause and breathe), the feel of the environment (pause), the fine points of the setting as they encircle you (pause), and soothing aromas or scents that allow you to feel calm (pause). In this moment, take pleasure in this image; create a memory of this relaxation to form in your mind, spreading to your muscles and tissues.

After a few moments, when you are ready, release the pain or areas of tension with an image of a round ball of light in any color that you would like to represent the pain. As you bring your awareness to this light, you are able to dim this light, slowly dimming the ball of light until it is smaller and smaller, releasing the pain and tension (breathe and be quiet for several minutes).

After 2–3 minutes and when ready, allow yourself to create a memory of this feeling of relaxation and comfort. Restfully focus your awareness on areas of your body that need healing. Send healing light to any areas with energy depletion, allowing

continues

continued

yourself to heal and send this feeling to smooth the progress of healing throughout your mind, body, and spirit.

Allow time for rest and integration of these images in your system. When returning to the environment, take deep breaths and stretch. Drink water. Assess the effects of the session. Repeat as desired.

TWELVE COPING STRATEGIES FOR STRESS MANAGEMENT

DR. MARTY DOWNEY

1. *Change your environment: Your five senses take in a great deal of information that you are not conscious of processing. If you find that the desk you are working at or the place that you are in most of the day has a great deal of distracting noises or irritable lights and sounds and smells, look around and see how you can make the environment friendlier to your senses. Change the lighting; add music, flowers, and fun pictures or photos.*

2. *Assert yourself: Stick up for your own needs without aggressiveness if you find that your choices are not your own or that you are building up feelings of resentment or anger because you feel taken for granted. Look to your own inner talk. Begin to make choices with your heart and mind, and tell others how you feel; no one can read your mind. It must come from you to make the changes that you feel are needed.*

3. *Change how you view things; change your mind: The key to stress reactions is recognition and awareness of thoughts that you have about any event. As you begin to expand the consciousness of your thought patterns, both negative and positive, you are sending positive thoughts to your mind, body, and spirit. These are the first steps in recovering from "toxic thinking." Stressful events can be viewed as challenges instead of threats. Think how you will feel*

when you have completed or finished the challenge, and then celebrate! Reflect on your inner dialogue; what you repeatedly say creates your reality and sends messages to your body that it might physically absorb and resonate. Take a moment to think of positive, supportive words and phrases in your inner dialogue that set your future health and success.

4. *Sit in silence every day: Our lives are filled with distractions. To clear our minds, we need to turn off the phone, television, computer, music, and other distractions and step away from chaos into silence. In these "silent moments," we can refresh and reenergize, so create your quiet place—a special corner, garden, calm spot. Take a deep breath and begin to clear your mind to create space for positive thoughts. Meditate, pray, and center yourself.*

5. *Organize your time: Learn to say "no" appropriately and "yes" to things that fit you. Exercise can fit into this schedule if you make it a priority. Write down your schedule and place a number to prioritize the things that need to be done today, those that can be done on other days, and those that are "nice to do." Be in control of the demands of your life by prioritizing and organizing.*

6. *Exercise: Regular exercise gives your body, mind, and spirit the boost they need to support you during stressful times and creates a strong, healthy lifestyle. It is an excellent outlet for the endorphin release that improves your mood and gives positive feelings of energy and euphoria. You can "tune in" to your body, mind, and spirit through exercise. Make this a priority, and it will become a truly healthy and rewarding ritual.*

7. *Nutrition: When you are under stress, do you maintain healthy nutrition? We might overeat or under-eat. Neither of these eating patterns is healthy. Next time you are on edge and feeling tense, note your eating patterns. What have you been eating and drinking? Replace the fast foods with foods that are whole, foods that come in their own packages. Fruits*

continues

continued

and vegetables come in their own package/peels if they are not processed (a potato is a whole food but potato chips are not!). Add a few of these whole foods to your intake each day. This will transform your stress eating and create more energy to take on stressful situations. Also, slow down when you are eating; eat mindfully. Look at the food before you eat it; take a moment to think of how long it took to prepare this food, and notice its texture, aroma, taste, and the feel in your mouth. Think of the process of eating with your health in mind.

8. *Rest: Create a healthy ritual at bedtime by making it clear to your body, mind, and spirit that you are going to rest. Shut off the computer 20 minutes before you go to bed. Sleep in an environment with few distractions. Calm down, take a bath, or read a book, listen to music, and place a pad of paper next to your bed to write down any thoughts that come into your mind as you are preparing for rest. Use relaxation techniques of imagery and visualization to begin the resting process. Sleep with intention and wake with purpose.*

9. *Learn to relax: Many forms of relaxation exist— massage, music therapy, imagery, meditation, prayer, yoga, pet therapy, and many more. Look for practitioners and instruction on how to use these techniques for relaxation.*

10. *Avoid overindulging or overmedicating: Drugs, alcohol, smoking, and binge eating place extra stress on your body to metabolize and process these toxic agents. The body is already trying very hard to adjust to the demands of the day. It works so hard for you to adapt during stress, so why would you place extra health hazards on top of the stress response? It is like driving without a seatbelt.*

11. *Develop a healthy support system: Find people in your life who believe in you and support you. Too many "energy vampires" around would love to steal your energy, so find others who love and celebrate YOU. Choose a person who is positive and gives you*

> *a warm feeling when you are with him or her. Every-*
> *one needs to have someone to rely on, and we should*
> *be someone whom others can rely on, too.*
>
> 12. *Laugh! Keep a sense of humor, take yourself lightly:*
>   *Studies show that people who look at life with a*
>   *twinkle in their eye and laugh at themselves have*
>   *lower blood pressure, less muscle tension, healthier*
>   *appetites, and fewer illnesses. Begin to look at life's*
>   *unintended funny moments, lighten up, and choose*
>   *moments that create calm through the challenges that*
>   *life gives you. Tell good jokes, giggle, guffaw, and*
>   *smile. Laughing 100 times a day can be as good as*
>   *exercising for 1 hour!*

Finishing Touches

Stress is a given in our lives. In the short term, stress can create a sense of alertness, vigilance, and might even give us "an edge." However, chronic and prolonged levels of heightened stress can have devastating effects. These increased stress levels can cause disruption in our usual activities and responsibilities. In some cases, high stress can result in uncivil behaviors. Because of the connections among stress, illness, and incivility, all of us need to nurture ourselves and to foster an environment of civility through stress-reduction and self-care.

CIVILITY TIP

Because stress is a major contributor to incivility and disruptive behavior, each of us needs to find and use stress-management strategies that work best for us. Try the 5-minute rule—select a physical exercise such as walking, jogging, biking—or if you are feeling particularly adventuresome, try strapping on the boxing gloves and hitting the heavy bags. If after 5 minutes you want to quit, so be it, but it is likely that you will feel so strong and confident that you will want to keep on going.

Chapter 12

Seeking and Keeping Civility in Nursing Education

It is time to break the fever of incivility and create a state of health in our academic and practice workplaces, and by extension, society at large.
–Cynthia Clark

In this final chapter, I want to write to you in a very personal way. I opened this book describing the sunrise moments and walks that start my day. With this chapter, the sun sets with an inspiration for each of us to invest in our own personal and collective pursuit of civility and to continue the conversation for fostering civility in nursing education and beyond.

As nurses, we understand and rely on the language of the discipline— so I ask you this, "Do you have your skilled and adept fingers on the pulse of your own civility? And if we conducted an MRI of your soul (or my soul), would we detect kindness and civility?"

All You Really Need to Know About Civility

This book opened with a variety of reflections on civility and incivility and encouraged readers to lead a more examined life—that despite our stressful work and life conditions, we must be self-aware of how our behaviors impact others. As Maxey (2011) reminds us, "Civility is the affirmation of the dignity of other human beings with whom we interact and in large part is a version of the Golden Rule" (p. 22). Conducting ourselves with civility and consideration can be challenging, especially in our fast-paced society and high-stress work environments, yet we must make civility a priority for our students, colleagues, practice partners, and ourselves. To do otherwise is to rob ourselves and others of a life well-lived. For all of us, civility is a choice—a decision to treat others in the way we want to be treated. In my faculty role, like Maxey (2011), my students frequently set a classroom norm to "abide by the Golden Rule"—this simple but often difficult-to-achieve adage is an uncomplicated and elegant way to navigate life. It reminds me of a conversation I had recently with a nurse educator from the Midwest. She said, "I think civility was captured in the book *All I Really Need to Know I Learned in Kindergarten*." I heartily agreed, and we engaged in a lively conversation about the profound and important lessons of kindergarten.

This beautifully and artfully written book was first published by Robert Fulghum in 1989. Fulghum suggests that we might know what is necessary to live an examined life, but living it is quite another matter and, to be sure, no picnic. This gifted author reminds us that wisdom is not necessarily found at the top of the graduate-school mountain but instead in the sandboxes of kindergarten. Some of Fulghum's wisdom includes sharing everything, playing fair, not hitting anyone, and saying you're sorry when you hurt somebody.

In utter simplicity, everything we really need to know to live a civil life is included in Fulghum's list somewhere—the Golden Rule, cleanliness, ecology, politics, and the circle of life. Simplicity notwithstanding, living by these tenets and choosing civility require deliberation and focus. It's not always easy, but then again, if it were easy, everyone would do it.

Fulghum's work has inspired me to create a list of my own civility wisdom (see the sidebar below).

DR. CLARK'S CIVILITY WISDOM (INSPIRED BY THE WORK OF ROBERT FULGHUM)

Practice forgiveness.

Express gratitude.

Affirm others.

Seek to live in a state of grace.

Respect the earth.

Make a difference.

Listen and be present.

Smile and spread goodwill.

Address unkindness.

Be kind to animals.

Exceed expectations.

Stand for something good.

Don't interrupt.

Be on time.

Avoid making assumptions.

Suspend judgment.

Don't butt in line.

Say please and thank you.

Put yourself in others' shoes.

Think before you speak.

This list of civility wisdom to some extent summarizes the essence of this book; like the elegance of poetry, it is the précis of the prose presented in the previous chapters, attempting to express what came before and providing the reader with an abridged version for living civility.

Often times, increased and prolonged levels of stress get in our way and cause us to act in ways that we might not otherwise act. Think about it—when you have behaved rudely toward another person (and we all have), the encounter likely occurred when you were stressed, rushed, tired, and maybe even hungry. Therefore, managing our stress, taking care of ourselves, and nurturing our minds, bodies, and spirits go a long way in creating and sustaining civility in our personal lives as well as our professional lives. In our world as nurse educators, stress is a given, and it will not be going away. Let's face it—nurses are in the business of life and death, and beyond that, we are responsible for students in the clinical settings where one mistake can be harmful, and in some cases, even fatal. Talk about stress!

So then, the real issue is not necessarily stress, but rather our ability to effectively cope with it. Whatever you are doing that brings you joy, keep doing it. My husband and our four dogs (all shelter pets; rejects that no one else really wants) often start our day by hiking through the high desert of southwest Idaho. The crisp nip of an autumn day, juxtaposed with the warming October sun, makes for an incredible stress buster. In our family, we often refer to our experiences in the outdoors as worshiping in the Cathedral of the Blue Dome—meaning that we marvel in the natural wonder that exists under a big, bold, wide-open sky. For us, being outdoors means restoration, renewal, and rekindling the spirit. It helps us de-clutter our minds, think more clearly, and rededicate ourselves to a meaningful life. Whatever it is that brings you contentment, especially after a particularly challenging day, do it, and keep doing it. You deserve it! And because we know that there is a definite connection between stress and incivility, taking care of ourselves and nurturing the spirit are foundational to living a purposeful life and fulfilling our commitment to fostering civility and interacting with kindness.

It is my fervent hope that offering a thoughtful gesture or simple act of kindness will never go out of style. Yet, so often, we fail to pause and acknowledge others amid the hectic, fast-paced flurry of our lives. In spring 2016, our youngest daughter graduated with her undergraduate degree. Brigadier General Erik C. Peterson, a highly decorated and distinguished commander of the U.S. Army Special Operations Aviation Command, delivered the commencement address. His military awards and decorations are many and impressive. I found Gen. Peterson's speech compelling, passionate, powerful, and deeply relevant to the ideals of service, advocacy, and civility. He challenged us to share our skills, talents, energy, and gifts to benefit others and contribute to the common good. He suggested we make service a habit and a lifestyle, not just a single act, and he strongly encouraged us to "endeavor to be kind."

Quoting Albert Schweitzer, he stated, "Constant kindness can accomplish much. As the sun makes ice melt, kindness causes misunderstanding, mistrust, and hostility to evaporate." He further noted that, along his 30-year military journey, he has witnessed firsthand the very best and the very worst of humanity. He observed: "Nothing has had a more profound, sustained, positive impact on me than the occasional, conspicuous act of kindness of my fellow man, and the simple pleasure and reward of being able to extend the same. Kindness and civility with its inherent power are all too often overlooked….Simple acts of kindness not only serve to counter the burdens and travails of the recipient, but are also known to improve the well-being of the giver. The impact of a [genuine act of kindness] can be profound, lasting, and positively viral."

This powerful, passionate, and brilliant speech touched me deeply. It was a rallying cry to continue the path I am on—to be an avid advocate for civility, respect, and yes, kindness. And not only that, but to raise awareness and challenge myself and others to become "civility champions" dedicated to improving the lives of individuals, teams, organizations, and yes, maybe even society.

Remember that kindness is a choice. Think about ways you touch the lives of others. Perhaps you have rescued a pet, or, as in our family's case, multiple pets. Maybe you hold the elevator for someone dashing to catch it, or pack an extra lunch for your child to share with a less fortunate friend or classmate. Maybe when others are gossiping about someone else, you are the first to jump in and speak well of that individual. Perhaps you've sent a letter to a relative or former teacher letting them know the positive impact they've had on your life.

Compliment others. Smile and greet them. At the bank or grocery store, offer your place in line to someone with fewer items or who seems to be in a hurry—or do it just because. If you see litter, pick it up and throw it away. Bring your partner coffee in bed. Include others in conversation, especially those who tend to be shy or quiet. At the Starbucks drive-thru, pay for the order of the person behind you.

These are just a few ideas. I'm sure many of you have countless ways to say thank you or extend a kind gesture to another. As Gen. Peterson reminds us, endeavor to be humble and kind. It really can make a difference in the lives of others. Maybe even our own.

Nurse Educators: Living Up to Our Promise

In this final chapter, I want to honor and pay tribute to nurse educators around the world who, each and every day, work hard to make a difference in the lives of others. Their tenacity and dedication inspire us and model the way. Year after year, nurses are named the most trusted profession in America—extolling nurses' honesty, high ethical standards, caring, and fierce patient advocacy. This sacred honor has been hard won, but what would happen if the public really knew what we know—that incivility is taking a terrible toll on nurses. We can and must do better.

In my travels, I am encouraged by the gains that we are making to lift the veil on this problem and, better yet, to take bold action to foster civility openly and in the nooks and crannies that our work takes us, because, as we all know, nurses are everywhere, working tirelessly every day at the bedside, in emergency departments, critical-care units, clinics, classrooms, and boardrooms, in cancer units, outpatient clinics, parishes, neighborhoods, barrios, villages, and in the streets where the toxicity of poverty and despair threaten our resolve. Around the world, nurses are fighting the good fight to bring healing and promise to those in the deserts, jungles, and war zones and in areas that seem just out of reach. With a blend of courage and grace, we are there.

Nurses advocate and care for the injured and the ill, the elderly and the infirm. We comfort the mentally ill and the homeless, providing care to those who have so little and who often need so much; administering to the dying to make their end-of-life care as painless and as peaceful as possible; delivering babies who represent the promise of a bright future and a new tomorrow; caring for the profoundly ill, tiny infant, a reluctant resident in the neonatal intensive care unit, and then watching that baby thrive, grow, and eventually go home. Nurse educators teach and foster student learning, and work tirelessly to prepare and educate our nursing workforce and to kindle the flame for practice, leadership, and activism. Nurses are consistently present to love the unlovable, to help the helpless, and to cultivate hope where hope sometimes seems impossible. As nurses, we have individually and collectively harnessed and galvanized our passion and purpose to improve the lives of others. Seeking, discovering, and then using our passion to create good in the world have long been the legacy and tradition of all nurses.

As members of the brotherhood and sisterhood of nursing, each of us must chart our own course and be clear about the future of our nursing practice and the principles that frame it. This requires thoughtful deliberation and the courage to lean into ambiguity while simultaneously experiencing the creative tension that exists between our current reality and our desired future. It calls for a close examination of our principles—principles like integrity and social justice, and civility—and daily habits, such as filling the reservoir of goodwill and keeping it as full as possible so that when we need to draw from that reservoir, it's sufficiently full. The course we are charting begins with our first nursing job and develops into a career through an organic process, and if we pay close attention and have a little bit of luck, we will discover our calling, one that fills us with a sense of renewal, fulfillment, accomplishment, and deep satisfaction.

Seeking Your Golden Moment

You might recall the description of my "golden moment," detailed in Chapter 5, when our supervisor gathered our crew in a spontaneously called meeting to acknowledge and celebrate that rare and special assembly of people fully dedicated to making a difference in the lives of others, a team of caring professionals who loved the kids entrusted to our care and each other. That golden moment is a deep and fond memory I still treasure today, years after that incredible time in my life. For those who have yet to experience your golden moment—seek it, grasp it tightly, and celebrate the joy! For those who are fortunate to have experienced or who are experiencing your golden moment, relish it and then share it with others. When nurses share their stories, the world listens.

Take the most recent Institute of Medicine (IOM) report (2011)—living proof of the nation and the world listening to nurses and, more importantly, calling on us to individually and collectively come together to lead the change to advance our nation's health. It is one of the most formidable reports ever generated for and on behalf of nurses. A nation turns to this noble profession of nursing with an unwavering belief and steadfast conviction that we can and will do it, that nurses can and will bring their "A game" and their considerable know-how to advance our nation's health.

As nurses, we are more than 3 million voices strong, the largest and most influential segment of the healthcare system. We are uniquely called upon to use not only our keen minds, science, and evidence to bring about change, but also to bring our humility, simple decency, caring, and civility to create and mobilize purposeful, transformational change. Ultimately, our purpose as members of the nursing profession is clear and intentional—to garner our collective wisdom, creativity, and hard work to improve the lives of others. The work and road ahead will be arduous, but we have others who have led the way—mentors who have helped us achieve lofty goals; who have unceasingly and unselfishly coached us, encouraged us, and believed in us; who have shared their knowledge with a spirit of generosity; and who have boldly led the way.

Our collective energy and combined commitment to nursing excellence is a definite force to be reckoned with as we foster civility near and far and lead the way in advancing our nation's health. So, proudly share your stories and experiences with others and use them as catalysts to create personal, organizational, and transformational change. When we relate and share our stories, we make meaning of and provide a rich texture and context for a life well-lived.

I encourage early-career nurses to seek out supportive mentors and urge experienced nurses to inspire and ignite the passion for nursing in our rising stars. As you begin to realize and achieve your passion and your purpose, unfortunately, you might encounter naysayers, individuals who seek to diminish your contributions, thwart your progress, and demean your ideas. Make every attempt to re-categorize these critics as "motivators" and reframe their discouragement to inspire action. They might not believe in you, but you must believe in yourselves and in nurses' combined ability to realize our purpose and vision for the future.

This purpose and vision can best be accomplished by aligning ourselves with positive role models who encourage and inspire us to reach our goals. We need to show gratitude, and then we need to "pay it forward" by modeling the way for others. Some days our path will be clear and our achievements heady; other times we might feel burdened and alone. At these times we must remind ourselves of our vision and purpose and do the work we were created to do. We can call upon words of wisdom from others, like the Bitterroot Salish tribal elder Debra Magpie Earling, who penned a poem titled "We Dance" and wrote,

We dance for our families

We dance for those who cannot dance

We dance for our babies and our elders

We dance in memory of all those who have left us and can no longer join us in the dance

So, when dancing becomes difficult, keep dancing

When your feet fall heavy on the ground—dance harder— Dance for your people, dance for all living things, and dance for yourself (1993)

As we all know, life is not a solo act, and none of us makes it alone. So much of what is good in my life—and perhaps yours—is a testimony to the power of positive mentorship (both personal and professional). I mentioned a saying in an earlier chapter (often attributed to Sir Isaac Newton) that goes, "If I have seen a little further it is by standing on the shoulders of giants." So to the many "giants" out there, we are grateful for your leadership and your courage to create and sustain a more civil society. So, continue to fuel your passion, fire up your purpose, and keep doing the work you were created to do. Seek and savor your golden moment, and dance like there's no tomorrow. To nurse educators everywhere, we salute you, we celebrate you, and, most of all, we thank you.

References

Achacoso, M. V. (2006). *"What do you mean my grade is not an A?" An investigation of academic entitlement, causal attributions, and self-regulation in college students* (Doctoral dissertation). University of Texas, Austin, TX.

Agency for Healthcare Research & Quality (AHRQ). (2016). *TeamSTEPPS national implementation.* Retrieved from http://teamstepps.ahrq.gov

Almost, J. (2006). Conflict within nursing work environments: Concept analysis. *Journal of Advanced Nursing, 53*(4), 444–453.

Altmiller, G. (2012). Student perceptions of incivility in nursing education: Implications for educators. *Nursing Education Perspectives, 33*(1), 15–20.

American Association of Colleges of Nursing (AACN). (2008). *The essentials of baccalaureate education for professional nursing practice.* Retrieved from http://www.aacn.nche.edu/education-resources/BaccEssentials08.pdf

American Association of Critical-Care Nurses (AACN). (2016). *AACN standards for establishing and sustaining healthy work environments: A journey to excellence* (2nd ed.). Retrieved from http://www.aacn.org/WD/HWE/Docs/HWEStandards.pdf

American College Health Association (ACHA). (2015, Fall). *National College Health Assessment student health survey.* Retrieved from http://www.acha-ncha.org/reports_ACHA-NCHAIIc.html

American Holistic Nurses Association (AHNA). (2016). *Holistic stress management for nurses.* Retrieved from http://www.ahna.org/Resources/Stress-Management

American Nurses Association (ANA). (2015a). *Code of ethics for nurses with interpretive statements.* Washington, DC: American Nurses Association.

American Nurses Association (ANA). (2015b, July 22). *Incivility, bullying, and workplace violence* [Position statement]. Retrieved from http://www. nursingworld.org/MainMenuCategories/WorkplaceSafety/Healthy-Nurse/ bullyingworkplaceviolence/Incivility-Bullying-and-Workplace-Violence. html

American Nurses Association (ANA). (2015c). *Nursing: Scope and standards of practice* (3rd ed.). Silver Spring, MD: Nursebooks.org.

American Nurses Association (ANA). (2016). *Healthy work environment.* Retrieved from http://www.nursingworld.org/MainMenuCategories/ WorkplaceSafety/Healthy-Work-Environment

American Nurses Credentialing Center (ANCC). (2016). *Forces of magnetism.* Retrieved from http://www.nursecredentialing.org/Magnet/ ProgramOverview/HistoryoftheMagnetProgram/ForcesofMagnetism

American Psychological Association (APA). (2016, March 10). *Stress in America: The impact of discrimination.* Retrieved from http://www.apa. org/news/press/releases/stress/2015/impact-of-discrimination.pdf

American Psychological Association (APA), Center for Organizational Excellence. (2015). *Psychologically healthy workplace awards, 2015.* Retrieved from http://www.apaexcellence.org/assets/general/2015-phwa- oea-magazine.pdf

Angelo, T. A., & Cross, K. P. (1993). *Classroom assessment techniques: A handbook for college teachers* (2nd ed.). San Francisco, CA: Jossey-Bass.

Arehart-Treichel, J. (2002, March 15). Mental illness on rise on college campuses. *Psychiatric News, 37*(6), 6–38. Retrieved from http:// psychnews.psychiatryonline.org/doi/full/10.1176/pn.37.6.0006

Associated Press-NORC Center for Public Affairs Research. (2016, April 15). *New survey shows Americans believe civility is on the decline.* Retrieved from http://www.apnorc.org/PDFs/Rudeness/APNORC%20Rude%20 Behavior%20Report%20%20PRESS%20RELEASE.pdf

Association of International Educators. (2010). *The changing landscape of global higher education.* Retrieved from http://www.nafsa.org/_/File/_/ positioning_brochure.pdf

Babenko-Mould, Y., & Laschinger, H. K. (2014). Effects of incivility in clinical practice settings on nursing student burnout. *International Journal of Nursing Education Scholarship, 11*(1), 145–154.

Bain, K. (2004). *What the best college teachers do.* Cambridge, MA: Harvard University Press.

Benegbi, S. (2012). *7 steps to achieving immediate calm confidence.* Retrieved from http://www.calmconfidence.com/7steps.asp

Benner, P., Sutphen, M., Leonard, V., & Day, L. (2010). *Educating nurses: A call for radical transformation.* San Francisco, CA: Jossey-Bass.

Bennis, W. G. (2009). *On becoming a leader.* New York, NY: Basic Books.

Bichsel, J. (June, 2013). *The state of e-learning in higher education: An eye toward growth and increased access* (Research report). Louisville, CO: EDUCAUSE Center for Analysis and research. Retrieved from https://net.educause.edu/ir/library/pdf/ers1304/ERS1304.pdf

Bigelow, B., & Arndt, M. (2005). Transformational change in health care: Changing the question. *Hospital Topics: Research and Perspectives on Health Care, 82*(2), 19–26.

Billings, D. M., & Halstead, J. A. (2016). *Teaching in nursing: A guide for faculty* (5th ed.). St. Louis, MO: Saunders Elsevier.

Blanchard, K. H. (1999). *The heart of a leader.* Tulsa, OK: Honor Books.

Boice, B. (1996). Classroom incivilities. *Research in Higher Education, 37*(4), 453–486. doi: 10.1007/BF01730110

Bonnel, W. E., & Vogel Smith, K. (2010). *Teaching technologies in nursing and the health professions: Beyond simulation and online courses.* New York, NY: Springer.

Boyer, E. L. (1990). *Scholarship reconsidered: Priorities of the professoriate.* Princeton, NJ: Carnegie Foundation for the Advancement of Teaching.

Brady, M. (2010). Healthy nursing academic work environments. *OJIN: The Online Journal of Issues in Nursing, 15*(1), Manuscript 6.

Braxton, J. M., & Bayer, A. E. (1999). *Faculty misconduct in collegiate teaching.* Baltimore, MD: Johns Hopkins University Press.

Braxton, J. M., & Bayer, A. E. (2004). *Addressing faculty and student classroom improprieties: New directions for teaching and learning, Vol. 99.* San Francisco, CA: Jossey-Bass.

Brookfield, S. (1990). *The skillful teacher.* San Francisco, CA: Jossey-Bass.

Brookfield, S. D. (1995). *Becoming a critically reflective teacher*. San Francisco, CA: Jossey-Bass.

Brookfield, S. D. (2006). The skillful teacher. Retrieved from https://static1. squarespace.com/static/5738a0ccd51cd47f81977fe8/t/5750ee6c04426212 4f3e31ce/1464921738561/The_Skillful_Teacher_Workshop_Packet.pdf

Carbone, E. (1999). Students behaving badly in large classes. *New Directions for Teaching and Learning, 77*(Spring), 35–43. doi: 10.1002/tl.7704

Carnegie Foundation for the Advancement of Teaching. (1990). *Campus life: In search of community*. Princeton, NJ: Author.

Cashman, K. (1998). *Leadership from the inside out: Seven pathways to mastery*. Provo, UT: Executive Excellence Publishers.

Cashman, K. (2008). *Leadership from the inside out: Becoming a leader for life*. San Francisco, CA: Berrett-Koehler Publishers.

Caspersen, D. (2014). *Changing the conversation: The 17 principles of conflict resolution*. New York, NY: Penguin Books.

Castronovo, M. A., Pullizzi, A., & Evans, S. (2016). Nurse bullying: A review and a proposed solution. *Nursing Outlook, 64*(3), 208–214. doi: 10.1016/j.outlook.2015.11.008

Center for American Nurses. (2008). *Lateral violence and bullying in the workplace*. Retrieved from http://www.mc.vanderbilt.edu/root/pdfs/ nursing/center_lateral_violence_and_bullying_position_statement_from_ center_for_american_nurses.pdf

The Chronicle of Higher Education. (July 20, 2015). What makes a great college? 8th annual survey. Retrieved from http://www.chronicle.com/ article/article-content/231649/

Ciulla, J. B. (2003). *The ethics of leadership*. Belmont, CA: Wadsworth/ Thomas Learning.

Cipriano, R. E. (2011). *Facilitating a collegial department in higher education: Strategies for success*. San Francisco: Jossey-Bass

Clark, C. M. (2006). *Incivility in nursing education: Student perceptions of uncivil faculty behavior in the academic environment* (Doctoral dissertation, University of Idaho). Retrieved from *Dissertation Abstracts International*. (AAT 3092571)

Clark, C. M. (2008a). The dance of incivility in nursing education as described by nursing faculty and students. *Advances in Nursing Science, 31*(4), E37–E54. doi: 10.1097/01.ANS.0000341419.96338.a3

Clark, C. M. (2008b). Faculty and student assessment and experience with incivility in nursing education. *Journal of Nursing Education, 47*(10), 458–465.

Clark, C. M. (2009). Faculty field guide for promoting student civility in the classroom. *Nurse Educator, 34*(5), 194–197. doi: 10.1097/NNE.0b013e3181b2b589

Clark, C. M. (2010). The sweet spot of civility: My story. *Reflections on Nursing Leadership, 36*(1). Retrieved from http://www.reflectionsonnursingleadership.org/Pages/Vol36_1_Clark.aspx

Clark, C. M. (2011). Pursuing a culture of civility: An intervention study in one program of nursing. *Nurse Educator, 36*(3), 98–102. doi: 10.1097/NNE.0b013e3182161238

Clark, C. M. (2012a). Fostering civility in nursing education and practice [Two-part series]. *Reflections on Nursing Leadership, 38*(4), Sigma Theta Tau International Part I—Students, jedi knights and the promise of civility. Retrieved from http://www.reflectionsonnursingleadership.org/Pages/Vol38_4_Clark_CivilityPart1.aspx

Clark, C. M. (2012b, June 26). The power of mentoring: My story [Web log post]. *Musing of the great blue*. Retrieved from http://musingofthegreatblue.blogspot.com/2012_06_01_archive.html

Clark, C. M. (2013). National study on faculty-to-faculty incivility: Strategies to promote collegiality and civility. *Nurse Educator, 38*(3), 98–102. doi: 10.1097/NNE.0b013e31828dc1b2

Clark, C. M. (2014). *National study on nursing student perceptions of stress, coping, and academic civility* (Unpublished manuscript).

Clark, C. M. (2016, April 4). When people behave badly: How to recover if you're the target [Web log post]. *Musing of the great blue*. Retrieved from http://musingofthegreatblue.blogspot.com/2016/04/when-people-behave-badly-how-to-recover.html

Clark, C.M. (2017). An evidence-based approach to integrate civility, professionalism, and ethical practice into nursing curricula. *Nurse Educator, 42*(3). doi:10.1097/NNE.0000000000000331

Clark, C. M., & Ahten, S. (2010). Beginning the conversation: The nurse educator's role in preventing incivility in the workplace. *RN Idaho, 33*(3), 1, 5–6.

Clark, C. M., & Ahten, S. M. (2011a, March 24). The downward spiral: Incivility in nursing [Interviewer: Laura A. Stokowski]. *Medscape Nursing.* Retrieved from http://www.medscape.com/viewarticle/739328

Clark, C. M., & Ahten, S. M. (2011b, August 19). Nurses: Resetting the civility conversation. *Medscape Nursing.* Retrieved from http://www.medscape.com/viewarticle/748104

Clark, C. M., Ahten, S. M., & Macy, R. (2012). Using problem-based learning scenarios to prepare nursing students to address incivility. *Clinical Simulation in Nursing, 9*(3), e75–e83. doi: http://dx.doi.org/10.1016/j.ecns.2011.10.003

Clark, C. M., Ahten, S. M., & Macy, R. (2014). Nursing graduates' ability to address incivility: Kirkpatrick's level-3 evaluation. *Clinical Simulation in Nursing, 10*(8), 425–431. doi: http://dx.doi.org/10.1016/j.ecns.2014.04.005

Clark, C. M., Ahten, S. M., & Werth, L. (2012). Cyber-bullying and incivility in an online learning environment, Part 2: Promoting student success in the virtual classroom. *Nurse Educator, 37*(5), 192–197. doi: 10.1097/NNE.0b013e318262eb2b

Clark, C. M., Barbosa-Leiker, C., Gill, L., & Nguyen, D. T. (2015). Revision and psychometric testing of the Incivility in Nursing Education (INE) survey: Introducing the INE-R. *Journal of Nursing Education, 54*(6), 306–315. doi: 10.3928/01484834-20150515-01

Clark, C. M., Belcheir, M., Strohfus, P., & Springer, P. J. (2012). Development and description of the Culture and Climate Assessment Scale. *Journal of Nursing Education, 51*(2), 75–80. doi: 10.3928/01484834-20111230-01

Clark, C. M., & Carnosso, J. (2008). Civility: A concept analysis. *Journal of Theory Construction & Testing, 12*(1), 11–15.

Clark, C. M., & Davis-Kenaley, B. L. (2011). Faculty empowerment of students to foster civility in nursing education: A merging of two conceptual models. *Nursing Outlook, 59*(3), 158–165. doi: 10.1016/j.outlook.2010.12.005

Clark, C. M., Farnsworth, J., & Landrum, R. E. (2009). Development and description of the Incivility in Nursing Education (INE) survey. *Journal of Theory Construction and Testing, 13*(1), 7–15.

Clark, C. M., Juan, C. M., Allerton, B. W., Otterness, N. S., Jun, W. Y., & Wei, F. (2012). Faculty and student perceptions of academic incivility in the People's Republic of China. *Journal of Cultural Diversity, 19*(3), 85–93.

Clark, C. M., & Kenski, D. (in press). Promoting civility in the operating room: An ethical imperative. *AORN Journal.*

Clark, C. M., Landrum, R. E., & Nguyen, D. (2013). Development and description of the Organizational Civility Scale (OCS). *Journal of Theory Construction and Testing, 17*(1), 11–17.

Clark, C. M., Nguyen, D., & Barbosa-Leiker, C. (2014). Student perceptions of stress, coping, relationships, and academic civility: A longitudinal study. *Nurse Educator, 39(4),* 170–174. doi: 10.1097/ NNE.0000000000000049

Clark, C. M., Olender, L., Cardoni, C., & Kenski, D. (2011). Fostering civility in nursing education and practice: Nurse leader perspectives. *Journal of Nursing Administration, 41*(7/8), 324–330. doi: 10.1097/ NNA.0b013e31822509c4

Clark, C. M., Olender, L., Kenski, D., & Cardoni, C. (2013). Exploring and addressing faculty-to-faculty incivility in nursing education: A national perspective and literature review. *Journal of Nursing Education, 52*(4), 211–218. doi: 10.3928/01484834-20130319-01

Clark, C. M., Sattler, V. P., & Barbosa-Leiker, C. (2016). Development and testing of the Healthy Work Environment Inventory (HWEI): A reliable tool for assessing work environment health and satisfaction. *Journal of Nursing Education, 55*(10), 555–562.

Clark, C. M., & Springer, P. J. (2007a). Incivility in nursing education: A descriptive study on definitions and prevalence. *Journal of Nursing Education, 46*(1), 7–14.

Clark, C. M., & Springer, P. J. (2007b). Thoughts on incivility: Student and faculty perceptions of uncivil behavior in nursing education. *Nursing Education Perspectives, 28*(2), 93–97.

Clark, C. M., & Springer, P. J. (2010). Academic nurse leaders' role in fostering a culture of civility in nursing education. *Journal of Nursing Education, 49*(6), 319–325. doi: 10.3928/01484834-20100224-01

Clark, C. M., Werth, L., & Ahten, S. (2012). Cyber-bullying and incivility in the online learning environment: Part 1: Addressing faculty and student perceptions. *Nurse Educator, 37*(4), 150–156. doi: 10.1097/ NNE.0b013e31825a87e5

Cockerell, L. (2008). *Creating magic: 10 common sense leadership strategies from a life at Disney.* New York, NY: Currency Doubleday.

Connelly, R. J. (2009). Introducing a culture of civility in first-year college classes. *The Journal of General Education, 58*(1), 47–64.

Covey, S. R. (1989). *The 7 habits of highly effective people.* New York, NY: Simon & Schuster.

Crigger, N., & Godfrey, N. (2014). From the inside out: A new approach to teaching professional identity formation and professional ethics. *Journal of Professional Nursing, 12*(5), 376–382. doi: 10.1016/j. profnurs.2014.03.004

Curtis, J., Bowen, I., & Reid, A. (2007). You have no credibility: Nursing students' experiences of horizontal violence. *Nursing Education in Practice, 7*(3), 156–163.

Dacanay, A., Vaughn, S., Orr, M., Andre, J., & Mort, K. (2015). Factors contributing to nursing distance education student success. *Journal of Nursing Education and Practice, 5*(2), 34–39. doi: 10.5430/jnep.v5n2p34

Dahlberg, L. L., & Krug, E. G. (2002). Violence—A global public health problem. In E. G. Krug, L. L. Dahlberg, J. A. Mercy, A. B. Zwi, & R. Lozano (Eds.), *World report on violence and health* (pp. 1–56). Geneva, Switzerland: World Health Organization.

Davenport, N., Schwartz, R. D., & Elliott, G. P. (1999). *Mobbing: Emotional abuse in the American workplace.* Ames, IA: Civil Society Publishing.

Day, L. (2011). Using unfolding case studies in a subject-centered classroom. *Journal of Nursing Education, 50*(8), 447–452. doi: 10.3928/01484834-20110517-03

De Gagne, J. C., Choi, M., Ledbetter, L., Kang, H. S., & Clark, C.M. (2016). An integrative review of cybercivility in health professions education. *Nurse Educator, 41*(5), 239–245. doi: 10.1097/ NNE.0000000000000264. Retrieved from https://www.ncbi.nlm.nih.gov/ pubmed/27022683

DeLesky, K. (2013). Professionalism. In J. F. Giddens (Ed.), *Concepts for nursing practice* (pp. 359–364). St. Louis, MO: Elsevier.

Del Prato, D. (2013). Students' voices: The lived experience of faculty incivility as a barrier to professional formation in associate degree nursing education. *Nurse Education Today, 33*(3), 286–290. doi: 10.1016/j. nedt.2012.05.030

Del Prato, D., Bankert, E., Grust, P., & Joseph, J. (2011). Transforming nursing education: A review of stressors and strategies that support students' professional socialization. *Advances in Medical Education and Practice, 2*, 109–116. doi: https://dx.doi.org/10.2147/AMEP.S18359

Doherty, C., Landry, H., Pate, B., & Reid, H. (2016). Impact of communication competency training on nursing students self-advocacy skills. *Nurse Educator, 41*(5), 252–255. doi: 10.1097/NNE.0000000000000274

Downey, M. (2006). *An investigation on education and use of complementary and alternative therapies by nurses in personal and professional practice* (Doctoral dissertation). University of Idaho, Moscow, ID.

Dumpel, H. (2010). Hospital magnet status: Impact on RN autonomy and patient advocacy. *National Nurse, 106*(3), 22–27.

Emry, R. A., & Holmes, O. (2005, Spring). *Civility: The value of valuing differences.* The Senate Forum, XX, No. 2, California State University, Fullerton, Academic Senate Forum.

Everytown for Gun Safety. (2016). *197 school shootings in America since 2013.* Retrieved from http://everytownresearch.org/school-shootings/

Farkas, S., & Johnson, J. (2002). *Aggravating circumstances: A status report on rudeness in America.* A report from public agenda prepared for the Pew Charitable Trusts. Retrieved from http://research.policyarchive.org/5628.pdf

Feldman, L. J. (2001). Classroom civility is another of our instructor responsibilities. *College Teaching, 49*(4), 137–140.

Fisher, R., Ury, W., & Patton, B. (1991). *Getting to yes: Negotiating agreement without giving in.* New York, NY: Penguin Books.

Fleming, N. (2012). *VARK learning styles inventory.* Retrieved from http://www.vark-learn.com

Forni, P. M. (2002). *Choosing civility: The twenty-five rules of considerate conduct.* New York, NY: St. Martin's Press.

Forni, P. M. (2008). *The civility solution: What to do when people are rude.* New York, NY: St. Martin's Press.

Frankl, V. E. (1959). *Man's search for meaning: An introduction to logotherapy* (3rd ed.). New York, NY: Simon & Schuster.

Freshman, B., & Rubino, L. (2002). Emotional intelligence: A core competency for health care administrators. *The Health Care Manager,* *20*(4), 1–9.

Fulghum, R. (1989). *All I really need to know I learned in kindergarten: Uncommon thoughts on common things.* New York, NY: Ivy.

Fuller, R. W. (2003). *Somebodies and nobodies: Overcoming the abuse of rank.* British Columbia, Canada: New Society Publishers.

Galbraith, M. W., & Jones, M. S. (2010). Understanding incivility in online teaching. *Journal of Adult Education, 39*(2), 1–10.

Gallup. (2016). *Honesty/ethics in professions.* Retrieved from http://www. gallup.com/poll/1654/honesty-ethics-professions.aspx

Garrison, D. R., & Akyol, Z. (2013). The community of inquiry theoretical framework. In M. G. Moore (Ed.), *Handbook of distance education* (3rd ed.) (pp. 104–120). New York, NY: Routledge.

Gehrke, P. M. (2012). *Engaging in learning together: A theory of undergraduate nursing students' political learning* (Unpublished doctoral dissertation). Boise State University, Boise, ID.

Giddons, J. F. (2013). *Concepts for nursing practice.* St. Louis, MO: Elsevier.

Gonzalez, V., & Lopez, E. (2001). The age of incivility: Countering disruptive behavior in the classroom. *American Association for Higher Education Bulletin, 55*(8), 3–6.

Griffin, M. (2004). Teaching cognitive rehearsal as a shield for lateral violence: An intervention for newly licensed nurses. *Journal of Continuing Education in Nursing, 35*(6), 257–263.

Griffin, M. (2010). *Creating a culture of mutual respect and strategies for change.* Program of the SUNY-IT, Iota Delta Teaching Symposium. Utica, NY.

Griffin, M., & Clark, C. M. (2014). Revisiting cognitive rehearsal as an intervention against incivility and lateral violence in nursing: 10 years later. *Journal of Continuing Education in Nursing, 45*(12), 535–542. doi: 10.3928/00220124-20141122-02

Guinness, O. (2008). *The case for civility: And why our future depends on it.* New York, NY: Harper Collins.

Hall, J. M. (2004). Dispelling desperation in nursing education. *Nursing Outlook, 52*(3), 147–154.

Hanson, M. F. (2000). *Classroom incivility: Management practices in large lecture course* (Doctoral dissertation, South Dakota State University). Dissertation Abstracts International.

Harper, J. (2013, March). Surviving workplace mobbing: Identify the stages. *Psychology Today*. Retrieved from http://www.psychologytoday.com/blog/beyond-bullying/201303/surviving-workplace-mobbing-identify-the-stages

Heinrich, K. T. (2006a). Joy-stealing games. *Reflections on Nursing Leadership, 32*(2). Retrieved from http://www.reflectionsonnursingleadership.org/Pages/Vol32_2_Heinrich.aspx

Heinrich, K. T. (2006b). Joy-stealing: How some nurse educators resist these faculty games. *Reflections on Nursing Leadership, 32*(3). Retrieved from http://www.reflectionsonnursingleadership.org/Pages/Vol32_3_Heinrich.aspx

Heinrich, K. T. (2007). Joy stealing: Ten mean games faculty play and how to stop the gaming. *Nurse Educator, 32*(1), 34–38.

Heinrich, K. T. (2010a). An optimist's guide for cultivating civility among academic nurses. *Journal of Professional Nursing, 26*(6), 325–331.

Heinrich, K. T. (2010b). Passionate scholarship 2001–2010: A vision for making academe safer for joyous risk-takers. *Advances in Nursing Science, 33*(1), E50–E64. doi: 10.1097/ANS.0b013e3181cd83ab

Heinrich, K. T. (2011). Take the civility challenge: How partnership practices can turn toxic workplaces terrific. *Nurse Educator, 36*(5), 224–227. doi: 10.1097/NNE.0b013e3182297c61

Heinrich, K. T., Clark, C. M., & Luparell, S. (2008). What are three words that turn competitions into collaborations? In K. T. Heinrich (Ed.), *A nurse's guide to presenting and publishing: Dare to share* (pp. 381–393). Sudbury, MA: Jones & Bartlett.

Hinduja, S., & Patchin, J. W. (2010). Bullying, cyberbullying, and suicide. *Archives of Suicide Research, 14*(3), 206–221.

Houshmand, M., O'Reilly, J., Robinson, S., & Wolff, A. (2012). Escaping bullying: The simultaneous impact of individual and unit-level bullying on turnover intentions. *Human Relations, 65*(7), 901–918.

How to use the Socratic Method in the classroom. (n.d.). Pedagogy in Action: The SERC portal for Educators. Retrieved from http://serc.carleton.edu/sp/library/socratic/fourth.html

Huss, J. A., Sela, O., & Eastep, S. (2015). A case study of online instructors and their quest for greater interactivity in their courses: Overcoming the distance in distance education. *Australian Journal of Teacher Education, 40*(4), 72–86.

Hutchings, P., & Shulman, L. S. (1999, September/October). The scholarship of teaching: New elaborations, new developments. *Change, 31*(5), 10–15. Retrieved from http://www.jstor.org/stable/40165542

Indiana University, Bloomington, Center for Survey Research. (2000, June 14). *A survey on academic incivility* (Preliminary report). Retrieved from http://spea.iupui.edu/documents/Incivility%20at%20IU.pdf

Institute of Medicine (IOM). (2003). *Health professions education: A bridge to quality.* Washington, DC: National Academies Press.

Institute of Medicine (IOM). (2011). *The future of nursing: Leading change, advancing health.* Washington, DC: National Academies Press. Retrieved from http://www.nap.edu/catalog.php?record_id=12956

International Council of Nurses (ICN). (2012). *Code of ethics for nurses.* Retrieved from http://www.icn.ch/about-icn/code-of-ethics-for-nurses

Interprofessional Education Collaborative Expert Panel. (2011). *Core competencies for interprofessional collaborative practice: Report of an expert panel.* Washington, DC: Interprofessional Education Collaborative.

Ironside, P. M., & Valiga, T. M. (2006). Creating a vision for the future of nursing education: Moving toward excellence through innovation. *Nursing Education Perspectives, 27*(3), 120–121.

Jenkins, S. D., Kerber, C. S., & Woith, W. M. (2013). An intervention to promote civility among nursing students. *Nursing Education Perspectives, 34*(2), 95–100.

Jonsen, A. R., Siegler, M., & Winslade, W. (2010). *Clinical ethics: A practical approach to ethical decisions in clinical medicine* (7th ed.). New York, NY: McGraw-Hill, Health Professions Division.

Kadison, R., & DiGeronimo, T. F. (2004). *College of the overwhelmed: The campus mental health crisis and what to do about it.* San Francisco, CA: Jossey-Bass.

Kerber, C., Woith, W. M., Jenkins, S. H., & Schafer Astroth, K. (2015). Perceptions of new nurses concerning incivility in the workplace. *The Journal of Continuing Education in Nursing, 46*(11), 522–527. doi: 10.3928/00220124-20151020-05

Kouzes, J. M., & Posner, B. Z. (2012). *The leadership challenge workbook* (3rd ed.). San Francisco, CA: John Wiley & Sons.

Language of Caring. (2016). *Model for caring feedback: Holding each other accountable.* Retrieved from http://www.languageofcaring.com/resource/model-for-caring-feedback-holding-each-other-accountable/

Lashley, F. R., & de Meneses, M. (2001). Student civility in nursing programs: A national study. *Journal of Professional Nursing, 17*(2), 81–86.

Lasiter, S., Marchiondo, L., & Marchiondo, K. (2012). Student narratives on faculty incivility. *Nursing Outlook, 60*(3), 121–126. doi: 10.1016/j.outlook.2011.06.001

Latham, J. R. (1995, January). Visioning: The concept, trilogy, and process. *Quality Progress, 28*(4), 65–68.

Levine, A., & Dean, D. R. (2012). *Generation on a tight rope: A portrait of today's college student.* San Francisco, CA: Jossey-Bass.

Lewis, P. S., & Malecha, A. (2011). The impact of workplace incivility on the work environment, manager skill, and productivity. *The Journal of Nursing Administration, 41*(1), 41–47.

Lipson, C. (2004). *Doing honest work in college: How to prepare citations, avoid plagiarism, and achieve real academic success.* Chicago, IL: University of Chicago Press.

Luparell, S. (2003). *Critical incidents of incivility by nursing students: How uncivil encounters with students affect nursing faculty* (Doctoral dissertation, University of Nebraska). Dissertation Abstracts International.

Luparell, S. (2004). Faculty encounters with uncivil nursing students: An overview. *Journal of Professional Nursing, 20*(1), 59–67.

Luparell, S. (2011). Incivility in nursing: The connection between academia and clinical settings. *Critical Care Nurse, 31*(2), 92–95.

Magpie Earling, D. (1993). We dance. In J. Peterson (Ed.), *Sacred encounters: Father DeSmet and the Indians of the Rocky Mountain West* Norman, OK: University of Oklahoma Press.

Marchiondo, K., Marchiondo, L. A., & Lasiter, S. (2010). Faculty incivility: Effects on program satisfaction of BSN students. *Journal of Nursing Education, 49*(11), 608–614. doi: 10.3928/01484834-20100524-05

Mathis, R. L., & Jackson, J. H. (2008). *Human resource management* (12th ed.). Mason, OH: Thomson/South-Western Publisher.

Maxey, K. (2011). *Civil business: Civil practice in corporations and society.* Evergreen, CO: Colorado Writing Services.

Maxfield, D., Grenny, J., Lavendro, R., & Groah, L. (2011). *The silent treatment: Why safety tools and checklists aren't enough to save lives.* Retrieved from www.silenttreatmentstudy.com

Mayer, J. D., Salovey, P., & Caruso, D. (2000). Models of emotional intelligence. In R. J. Sternberg (Ed.), *The handbook of intelligence* (pp. 396–420). New York, NY: Cambridge University Press.

Mayne, L., & Wu, Q. (2011). Creating and measuring social presence in online graduate courses. *Nursing Education Perspectives, 32*(2), 110–114.

Mayo Clinic. (2015, September 17). *Job burnout: How to spot it and take action.* Retrieved from http://www.mayoclinic.org/healthy-lifestyle/adult-health/in-depth/burnout/art-20046642

McElveen, N. M., Leslie, P., & Malotky, D. (2006). Ethical issues in faculty conflict. *Teaching Ethics: The Journal of the Society for Ethics across the Curriculum, 7*(1), 33–56.

Miller, B. C. (n.d.). *Holding others accountable is SIMPLE.* Retrieved from http://communicoltd.com/Resources/Articles/Building-and-Sustaining-a-Service-Culture/Holding-Others-Accountable.aspx

Morrissette, P. J. (2001). Reducing incivility in the university/college classroom [Electronic version]. *International Electronic Journal for Leadership in Learning, 5*(4), 1–12.

Mott, J. (2014). Undergraduate nursing student experiences with faculty bullies. *Nurse Educator, 39*(3), 143–148. doi: 10.1097/NNE.0000000000000038

National Council of State Boards of Nursing (NCSBN). (2011, August). *White paper: A nurse's guide to the use of social media.* Retrieved from https://www.ncsbn.org/Social_Media.pdf

National League for Nursing (NLN). (2005). *Core competencies of nurse educators with task statements.* Retrieved from http://www.wgec.org/resources/art/nursing-core-competencies.pdf

National League for Nursing (NLN). (2006a). *The healthful work environment tool kit.* Retrieved from http://www.nln.org/docs/default-source/professional-development-programs/healthful-work-environment-toolkit.pdf?sfvrsn=2

National League for Nursing (NLN). (2006b). Mentoring of nurse faculty [Position Statement]. *Nursing Education Perspectives, 27*(2), 110–113.

Nick, J. M., Delahoyde, T. M., Del Prato, D., Mitchell, C., Ortiz, J., Ottley, C.,...Siktberg, L. (2012). Best practices in academic mentoring: A model for excellence. *Nursing Research and Practice,* 1–9. doi: 10.1155/2012/937906

Nilson, L. B. (2003). *Teaching at its best: A research-based resource for college instructors* (2nd ed.). San Francisco, CA: Jossey-Bass.

Northouse, P. G. (2012). *Introduction to leadership: Concepts and practice* (2nd ed.). Thousand Oaks, CA: SAGE Publishers Inc.

Olender-Russo, L. (2009). Creating a culture of regard: An antidote for workplace bullying. *Creative Nursing, 15*(2), 75–81.

Osatuke, K., Moore, S. C., Ward, C., Dyrenforth, S. R., & Belton, L. (2009). Civility, Respect, Engagement in the Workforce (CREW): Nationwide organization development intervention at Veterans Health Administration. *Journal of Applied Behavioral Science, 45*(3), 384–410. doi: 10.1177/0021886309335067

Oster, C. A., & Braaten, J. S. (2016). *High reliability organizations: A healthcare handbook for patient safety and quality.* Indianapolis, IN: Sigma Theta Tau International.

Palmer, P. J. (1998). *The courage to teach: Exploring the inner landscape of a teacher's life.* San Francisco, CA: Jossey-Bass.

Parker-Pope, T. (2005, July 19). Stress and your waistline: Gaining belly fat may be body's way of coping. *The Wall Street Journal.* Retrieved from http://www.wsj.com/articles/SB112172706650488801

Pearson, C., & Porath, C. (2009). *The cost of bad behavior: How incivility is damaging your business and what to do about it.* New York, NY: Penguin Group.

Pisanos, D. (2011). *The leader within: Integral leadership.* Presented at the Nurse Leaders of Idaho Statewide Conference, Boise, ID.

Porath, C., & Pearson, C. (2013, January–February). The price of incivility: Lack of respect hurts morale and the bottom line. *Harvard Business Review,* 115–121.

Quality and Safety Education for Nurses (QSEN). (2016). *Quality and safety competencies.* Retrieved from http://qsen.org/competencies/

Rieck, S., & Crouch, L. (2007). Connectiveness and civility in online learning. *Nursing Education in Practice, 7*(6), 425–432.

Science Education Resource Center at Carleton College. (2016). *How to use just-in-time teaching. Starting point: Teaching entry level geoscience.* Retrieved from http://serc.carleton.edu/introgeo/justintime/how.html

Senge, P. M. (1990). *The fifth discipline: The art and practice of the learning organization.* New York, NY: Doubleday Currency.

Showkeir, J., & Showkeir, M. (2008). *Authentic conversations: Moving from manipulation to truth and commitment.* San Francisco, CA: Berrett-Koehler Publishers.

Shulman, L. (2011). The scholarship of teaching and learning: A personal account and reflection. *International Journal for the Scholarship of Teaching and Learning, 5*(1). Retrieved from http://http://digitalcommons.georgiasouthern.edu/cgi/viewcontent.cgi?article=1249&context=ij-sotl

Sistare, C. T. (2004). *Civility and its discontents: Essays on civic virtue, tolerance, and cultural fragmentation.* Lawrence, KS: University Press of Kansas.

Smith, T. C. (2005). Fifty-one competencies for online instruction. *The Journal of Educators Online, 2*(2), 1–18.

Spence-Laschinger, H. K., Wong, C. A., Cummings, G. G., & Grau, A. L. (2014). Resonant leadership and workplace empowerment: The value of positive organizational cultures in reducing workplace incivility. *Nursing Economic$, 32*(1), 5–15.

Springer, P. J., Clark, C. M., Strohfus, P., & Belcheir, M. (2012). Using transformational change to improve organizational culture and climate in a school of nursing. *Journal of Nursing Education, 51*(2), 81–88. doi: 10.3928/01484834-20111230-02

Stanford School of Medicine. (2016). *Interactive learning.* Retrieved from http://med.stanford.edu/smili/interactive-learning/index.html

Sullivan, E. J. (2013). *Becoming influential: A guide for nurses* (2nd ed.). Boston, MA: Pearson Education.

Suplee, P. D., Lachman, V. D., Siebert, B., & Anselmi, K. K. (2008). Managing nursing student incivility in the classroom, clinical setting, and on-line. *Journal of Nursing Law, 12*(2), 68–77.

The Joint Commission (TJC). (July 9, 2008). *Sentinel Event Alert, Issue 40: Behaviors that undermine a culture of safety.* Retrieved from http://www. jointcommission.org/sentinel_event_alert_issue_40_behaviors_that_ undermine_a_culture_of_safety/

Thomas, S. P. (2003). Handling anger in the teacher-student relationship. *Nursing Education Perspective, 24*(1), 17–24.

Trépanier, S., Fernet, C., Austin, S., & Boudrias, V. (2016). Work environment antecedents of bullying: A review and integrative model applied to registered nurses. *International Journal of Nursing Studies, 55,* 85–97. doi: 10.1016/j.ijnurstu.2015.10.001

Tuckman, B. W. (1965). Developmental sequence in small groups. *Psychological Bulletin, 63*(6), 384–399.

Twale, D. J., & De Luca, B. M. (2008). *Faculty incivility: The rise of the academic bully culture and what to do about it.* San Francisco, CA: Jossey-Bass.

Vessey, J. A., DeMarco, R. F., Gaffney, D. A., & Budin, W. (2009). Bullying of staff registered nurses in the workplace: A preliminary study for developing personal and organizational strategies for transformation of hostile to healthy workplace environments. *Journal of Professional Nursing, 25,* 299–306.

Vincent, P. F. (2006). *Restoring school civility.* Greensboro, NC: Character Development Group.

Wankel, L. A., & Wankel, C. (Eds.). (2012). *Misbehavior online in higher education.* Bingley, UK: Emerald Group Publishing.

Weber Shandwick & Powell Tate (2013). *Civility in America 2013.* Retrieved from http://www.webershandwick.com/uploads/news/files/Civility_in_ America_2013_Exec_Summary.pdf

Weber Shandwick & Powell Tate (2014). *Civility in America 2014.* Retrieved from http://www.webershandwick.com/uploads/news/files/civility-in- america-2014.pdf

Weber Shandwick & Powell Tate. (2016). *Civility in America 2016.* Retrieved from https://www.webershandwick.com/news/article/civility-in-america- 2016-us-facing-a-civility-crisis

Weick, K., & Sutcliffe, K. (2007). *Managing the unexpected: Resilient performance in an age of uncertainty.* San Francisco, CA: Jossey-Bass.

Weil, A. (2011). *Spontaneous happiness: Your 8-week plan to a lifetime of emotional well-being.* New York, NY: Little, Brown and Company.

Westhues, K. (2004). *The envy of excellence: Administrative mobbing of high-achieving professors.* Lewiston, NY: Edwin Mellen Press.

Wheatley, M. J. (1994). *Leadership and the new science: Learning about organization from an orderly universe.* San Francisco, CA: Berrett-Koehler Publishers.

Woods, M. S. (2010). *Civil leadership: The final step to achieving safety, quality, innovation, and profitability in health care.* Oakbrook Terrace, IL: Joint Commission Resources.

Workplace Bullying Institute. (2014, February). *2014 WBI U.S. workplace bullying survey.* Retrieved from http://www.workplacebullying.org/wbiresearch/wbi-2014-us-survey/

Yoder-Wise, P. S. (2015). *Leading and managing in nursing* (6th ed.). St. Louis, MO: Elsevier/Mosby Publishers.

Younger, R. F., & Ahern, T. C. (2015). Is a quality course a worthy course? Designing for value and worth in online courses. *Online Journal of Distance Learning Administration, 18*(1).

Index

Resources for